ORGAN DONATION
AND TRANSPLANTATION

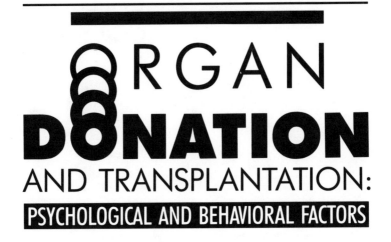

ORGAN DONATION AND TRANSPLANTATION:
PSYCHOLOGICAL AND BEHAVIORAL FACTORS

EDITED

BY

JAMES
SHANTEAU

AND

RICHARD
JACKSON
HARRIS

American Psychological Association

First printing June 1990
Second printing July 1992

Published by
American Psychological Association
750 First Street, NE
Washington, DC 20002

Copies may be ordered from
APA Order Department
P.O. Box 2710
Hyattsville, MD 20784

Designed by Paul M. Levy
Typeset by BG Composition, Baltimore, MD
Printed by Edwards Brothers, Inc., Ann Arbor, MI
Technical editing and production coordinated by
Valerie Montenegro and Theodore J. Baroody

Library of Congress Cataloging-in-Publication Data

Organ donation and transplantation : psychological and behavioral
factors / James Shanteau and Richard Jackson Harris, editors.
p. cm.
    Based on a conference held in Manhattan, KS, in 1988.
ISBN 1-55798-079-9 (cloth; acid-free paper)
    1. Donation of organs, tissues, etc.—Psychological aspects—
Congresses.   2. Transplantation of organs, tissues, etc.—
Psychological aspects—Congresses.
    I. Shanteau, James. II. Harris, Richard Jackson.
    [DNLM: 1. Organ Procurement—methods—congresses.   2. Tissue
Donors—psychology—congresses.   3. Transplantation—congresses. WO 660 0645]
RD129.5.074 1990   362.1'783'019—dc20   90-338

Printed in the United States of America.

CONTENTS

CONTRIBUTORS

Helen Levine Batten, *Brandeis University*
Russell W. Belk, *University of Utah*
Eugene Borgida, *University of Minnesota*
Cynthia Conner, *University of Minnesota*
Gaylord Cummins, *Tulane University*
Karen F. A. Fox, *Santa Clara University*
Kenneth R. Hammond, *University of Colorado*
Richard Jackson Harris, *Kansas State University*
Dick J. Hessing, *Eramus University Rotterdam and Leyden University*
John David Jasper, *University of Iowa*
Keren Ami Johnson, *Old Dominion University*
Herbert M. Lefcourt, *University of Waterloo*
Kimberly A. Linin, *Kansas State University*
Kirsten Lombard, *University of Minnesota*
Lola Lopes, *University of Wisconsin*
Patrick J. McGrath, *Dalhousie University*
Pat McIntyre, *University of North Carolina at Charlotte*
Barbara E. Nolan, *University of Ottawa*
Kenneth A. Perkins, *University of Pittsburgh*
Jane Allyn Piliavin, *University of Wisconsin—Madison*
David J. Schneider, *Rice University*
James Shanteau, *Kansas State University*
Robert Shepherd, *University of Waterloo*
Roberta G. Simmons, *University of Pittsburgh*
John J. Skowronski, *Ohio State University at Newark*
Stacy A. Smith, *University of Texas at Arlington*
Vinod K. Thukral, *Tulane University*

FOREWORD

Federal research agencies stopped regularly supporting investigator-initiated "state-of-the-art" research conferences in scientific psychology well over a decade ago. Yet, over that same period, scientific psychology has continued to grow—as well as to diversify into many new areas. Thus, there have been relatively few opportunities for investigators in new and cutting-edge research areas to convene in special settings to discuss their findings.

The American Psychological Association (APA), as part of its continuing efforts to enhance the dissemination of scientific knowledge in psychology, undertook a number of new initiatives designed to foster scientific research and communication. In particular, the APA Science Directorate, in 1988, initiated the Scientific Conferences Program.

The APA Scientific Conferences Program provides university-based psychological researchers with seed monies essential to organizing specialty conferences on critical issues in basic research, applied research, and methodological issues in psychology. Deciding which conferences to support involves a competitive process. An annual call for proposals is issued by the APA Science Directorate to solicit conference ideas. Proposals from all areas of psychological research are welcome. They are then reviewed by qualified psychologists, who forward substantive suggestions and funding recommendations to the Science Directorate. At each stage, the criteria used to determine which conferences to support include relevance, timeliness, and comprehensiveness of the topics, and qualifications of the presenters. In 1988, seven conferences were funded under this APA Science Directorate program's sponsorship, and six conferences were funded in 1989. We expect to fund six more in 1990, at an annual overall program expense of $90,000 to $100,000.

The APA Scientific Conferences Program has two major goals. The first is to provide, by means of the conferences, a broad view of specific topics (and, when appropriate, to provide for interdisciplinary participation). The second goal is to assure timely dissemination of the findings presented by publishing a series of carefully crafted scholarly volumes based, in part, on each conference. Thus, the information reaches the audiences at each conference as well as the broader psychological and scientific communities. This enables psychology and related fields to benefit from the most current research on a given topic.

This volume presents findings reported at the October 1988 conference, "Psychological Research on Organ Donation." The psychological issues involved in organ donation are highly specialized and represent a fascinating area of research that touches on many concerns in psychology: value systems, perceptions of self and others, the impact of societies' expectations and standards on individuals' decisions, the nature of decision making under pressure, and other issues. Basic and applied researchers from several fields came together at the conference, taking the first step in developing a new interdisciplinary research area.

This volume is representative of what we at the American Psychological Association believe will be a number of exceptional volumes that give readers a broad sampling of the diverse and outstanding research now being done in scientific psychology. We hope you will enjoy and be stimulated by this book and the many others to come.

A list of the conferences funded through this program follows:

Researching Community Psychology: Integrating Theories and Methodologies, September 1988
Psychological Well-Being in Nonhuman Captive Primates, September 1988
Psychological Research on Organ Donation, October 1988
Arizona Conference on Sleep and Cognition, January 1989
Socially Shared Cognition, February 1989
The Role of Experience in Modifying Taste and Its Effects on Feeding, April 1989
Perception of Structure, May 1989
Suggestibility of Children's Recollections, June 1989
Best Methods for the Analysis of Change, October 1989
Conceptualization and Measurement of Organism–Environment Interaction, November 1989
Cognitive Bases of Musical Communication, April 1990
Conference on Hostility, Coping/Support, and Health, November 1990
Psychological Testing of Hispanics, February 1991
Study of Cognition: Conceptual and Methodological Issues, February 1991

Gary R. VandenBos, PhD
Acting Executive Director
Science Directorate, APA

Virginia E. Holt
Manager, Scientific Conferences Program
Science Directorate, APA

CHAPTER 1

WHY PSYCHOLOGICAL RESEARCH ON ORGAN DONATION?

JAMES SHANTEAU AND RICHARD JACKSON HARRIS

This volume is an outgrowth of a conference held in Manhattan, Kansas, on October 2–4, 1988. That conference, "Psychological Research on Organ Donation," brought together researchers studying the problem of increasing organ donation in the United States, Canada, and Europe from a psychological perspective. To our knowledge, this was the first time such a meeting had occurred. Although the problems of organ transplantation have been widely studied and discussed from medical and ethical perspectives, the psychological focus has been neglected. Various investigators have examined behavioral issues, but there has been little communication or interaction among these researchers. The Manhattan conference and this book represent the only instances in which reports of such research have been assembled in one place.

THE DONOR ORGAN SHORTAGE

One of the marvels of modern medical technology is organ transplantation. Organs such as the kidney and the cornea are now transplanted with relative frequency. With one-year success rates approaching 90 percent or more (Sipes, 1987), such transplants are becoming routine (Hostetler, 1987). Moreover, the success rates for more difficult transplants, such as hearts and livers, have been steadily rising (U.S. Department of Health and Human Services, 1986). Thus, the technology of transplantation has developed rapidly as a life-saving procedure and promises to continue to improve.

A major roadblock, however, has been the inability to deliver the technology of transplantation to many patients in need. This is not due to a lack of skilled surgeons or even of money but rather to a shortage of organs available for transplantation. In part, the shortfall reflects an increase in the number of patients who might benefit from a transplant, due to better screening and improved immunosuppressant drugs (Caplan, 1984). The major reason for the shortage, however, is simply a lack of sufficient donors.

The ramifications of this shortage are tragic. In 1980 alone, approximately 14,000 people died because they did not receive needed heart transplants (Evans, Manninen, Gersh, Hart, & Rodin, 1984). The American Council on Transplantation estimated that there were 13,000 patients needing a kidney transplant on any given day in 1988 (Clark, Robinson, & Wickelgren, 1988). The need for other organs such as pancreas, liver, bone marrow, corneas, lungs, and skin, is also high, with around 10,000 people waiting for organs to become available (U.S. Department of Health and Human Services, 1988). Potential transplant recipients may wait for years, if they survive, before a suitable donor organ can be found. Unfortunately, the longer the delay, the greater the probability of medical complications.

These shortages do not appear to be due to lack of potential organs that are suitable for donation. One estimate concluded that only about 3,000 out of an estimated 23,000 organs that could be donated were in fact donated (Warmbrodt & Koch, 1985). Even a modest increase in the rate of donation would go a long way toward reducing this shortage because a single donor can provide over a dozen viable organs and tissues for transplantation. The central question is: Why are there so few decisions to donate?

One common answer in the medical literature is that lack of knowledge about the need for donors is responsible for the shortage. Accordingly, considerable effort has been made in recent years to increase awareness, even sympathy, regarding the plight of potential organ recipients (e.g., Baldwin, 1987; Greenfield, 1988; Gunby, 1983; Jones, 1988; Kalter, 1986; Krasner & Bailey, 1986; Thukral & Cummins, 1987). Surveys conducted by behavioral researchers, however, have shown consistently that almost everyone is aware of the need for organs (Manninen & Evans, 1985; Evans & Manninen, 1988). In studies of more than 800 residents of Kansas and Ohio, for example, almost 99 percent reported being aware of the shortage of donated organs (McIntyre et al., 1987; Skowronski, 1987). Moreover, most respondents indicated that they were sympathetic to the needs of potential recipients. Therefore, the shortage of organ donors does not appear to be due to a lack of knowledge or an absence of empathy (Barnett, Klassen, McMinimy, & Schwarz, 1987).

We believe that an important part of the answer to the organ shortage will come from a better understanding of the psychological processes involved in agreeing to organ donation. That is, reluctance to donate is due not to lack of knowledge but rather to unstated motivations, perceived risks, and unarticulated fears about donation (Fraumon & Miles, 1987; Hessing & Elffers, 1986; McIntyre et al., 1987; Prottas, 1983). We are convinced, therefore, that there is a pressing need for psychological research on the decision to donate organs.

Several distinct areas of psychology have actual or potential contributions to make in understanding the problem of obtaining organ donations. Researchers concerned with this issue can be found in almost every subfield of psychology. Consequently, the publications on organ donation that have appeared are widely scattered in the professional literature. This diversity exists partly because many of the psychologists studying the problem are working in nonpsychology positions, such as medical schools, marketing departments, or policy and administrative positions. There are also researchers trained in other disciplines, such as sociology or political science, who are currently doing what is essentially psychological research. As a result, the literature is largely unconnected and noncumulative. Despite these difficulties, various subfields of psychology have shown the potential for producing important insights into organ donation behavior. To illustrate, we will describe some contributions previously made by various subareas of psychology.

INSIGHTS FROM DIFFERENT AREAS OF PSYCHOLOGY

Helping Behavior and Altruism

The psychological literature on helping behavior includes examinations of the conditions under which people will help others and at what cost to themselves they will do so (Barnett, 1987; Eisenberg, 1982; Rushton & Sorrentino, 1981). Organ donation is a particularly interesting topic from the perspective of helping behavior (Sojka, 1985). On the one hand, becoming a living kidney donor represents a very generous but potentially risky way of helping. On the other hand, signing an organ donor card involves little or no immediate cost, with direct benefits never to be experienced by the donor. Agreeing as a next of kin to donate a deceased loved one's organs is a type of helping behavior necessarily occurring under conditions of extreme stress, emotional pain, and time pressure; this act, however, may become a part of the process of healing that pain.

Some research has been done on organ donation as helping behavior. Several studies have found that people's expressed motives for donating organs are primarily altruistic and other-oriented (Cleveland, 1975; Fellner & Marshall, 1981; Moores, Clarke, Lewis, & Mallick, 1976; Prottas, 1983). However, a more experimental approach found that potential donors responded more positively to a persuasive communication emphasizing benefits to themselves rather than one emphasizing benefits to others (Barnett, Klassen, McMinimy, & Schwarz, 1987).

Health Psychology

With the recent emphasis on the mind–body interaction, psychologists increasingly have examined biological correlates of behavior, and medical practitioners now consider psychological aspects of illness. In this context, taking a holistic approach to organ donation seems natural. The difficulties of increasing organ donation present an enormous medical problem to which psychology can speak.

Perkins (1987) carefully analyzed the current status of psychological research on organ donation and suggested several directions for future research. Parallel to our position, Perkins, as well as Olbrisch (1989), argued that psychology has much more to contribute than it has so far.

Judgment and Decision Making

The decision to become an organ donor, or to donate the organs of a next of kin, may be seen as a cognitive question of how information is sought, evaluated, and combined. According to this view, the keys to understanding organ donation are to analyze what factors influence the decision and to determine how these factors are integrated. Research by Wilms, Kiefer, Shanteau, and McIntyre (1987), for instance, revealed that donation decisions are largely affectively based. "Organ donors think little about their behavior. They donate because it 'feels right' " (p. 341). The psychological components of this feeling, however, have yet to be investigated.

The role that risk plays is often a crucial component in real-world decision behavior (Anderson, Deane, Hammond, McClelland, & Shanteau, 1981). Although there has been little empirical research relating risk to donation behavior, Shanteau (1986) suggested that a major reason for reluctance to donate organs may be perceived risk and unarticulated fears. A direct assessment of these risks, similar to analyses in other domains of uncertainty, may prove fruitful.

Social Psychology of Attitude Change

The social psychological study of attitudes and attitude change is clearly relevant to the issue of organ donation. Several studies of attitudes toward organ donation have found widely favorable attitudes toward the concept, but a low rate of signing organ donor cards (Corlett, 1985; Manninen & Evans, 1985; McIntyre et al., 1987; Moores et al., 1976; Prottas, 1983). Theory and constructs from social psychology (e.g., dissonance theory, attribution theory, and social schemas) offer intellectual tools useful in examining this inconsistency.

In terms of attitude change, there is great potential for campaigns to educate people about the need for organ donations and to persuade them to become donors. For several reasons, however, this is a difficult issue to study. People generally agree with the need and the concept much more readily than they agree to become donors themselves. Also, the discomfort of thinking about death and facing the prospect of one's own mortality can be a tremendous psychological barrier to signing a donor card.

The extreme emotional stress surrounding the decision to donate the organs of a next of kin makes it very difficult to study attitude change. Although this process is obviously inappropriate to simulate completely in the psychological laboratory, some field studies and observations have identified several important factors. These include the presence of supportive others, allowing the survivors time to absorb the shock of the death, and the sensitivity of the approach to the family (Bart et al., 1981; Fulton, Fulton, & Simmons, 1977; Haney, 1973;

Manning & McCabe, 1986). The most effective appeals are those that (a) provide needed information in a sensitive and tactful manner and (b) refute misconceptions about organ donation (Nuckolls, 1989; Parisi & Katz, 1986; Winkel,1984; Youngner et al., 1985).

Individual Differences

Some pronounced individual differences have been noted in the willingness to donate organs. Black people are less likely than White people to agree to become organ donors, although the need among the former is at least as high as in the White population (Callender, 1987; Hosten, 1987; Pollak, Prusak, Wiberg, & Mozes, 1986). Hispanics are less likely than Anglos to consent to donate the organs of a next of kin (Johnson et al., 1988; Perez, Matas, & Tellis, 1988). People of higher socioeconomic status (SES) are more likely to agree to become donors than those of lower SES; however, disproportionately more of the latter become actual donors, especially as a result of motor vehicle accidents (Manninen & Evans, 1985). Isolating the differences attributable to racial and ethnic groups and SES remains for future research, however. In terms of gender differences, several studies focusing on other issues have also revealed interesting male–female differences (e.g., Wilms et al., 1987).

Personality psychology may contribute by identifying distinguishing characteristics of actual and potential donors. Belk and Austin (1986), for instance, found that people who were more materialistic and for whom body organs were more central to their sense of self were less willing than others to donate organs. Royster, Tetreault, and Shanteau (1987) reported that people with higher death anxiety were less willing to become organ donors or to engage in other activities that presuppose death, such as preparing a will. How all these variables fit together, however, has yet to be investigated.

Legal Psychology

Psychology can provide important input to the development of proposed laws designed to encourage organ donation within acceptable philosophical and legal boundaries. The most common procedural change proposed is a required request for organ donation (Andersen & Fox, 1988; Francisco, 1987; Martyn, Wright, & Clark, 1988; Weedn & Leveque, 1988). The public's reactions to the concept of required request, however, have yet to be investigated.

Another issue concerns the mandatory information offered to potential donors. Such material could be designed to counteract misconceptions and reservations that act as psychological barriers to consent. If motivations to donate or not to donate were better understood, more effective appeals could be constructed (Barnett et al., 1987).

Social Marketing

Social marketing has recently blossomed as a major field of marketing (Barach, 1984; Bloom & Novelli, 1981; Fox & Kotler, 1980; Guy & Patton, 1989;

Rothschild, 1979). Marketing and management approaches to identifying populations and to "selling" the concept of organ donation have been offered (Pessemier, Bemmaor, & Hanssens, 1977; Thukral & Cummins, 1987). Still, most of the publicity campaigns dealing with organ donation have stressed medical issues or anecdotal case studies.

In comparison, models from other public health marketing promotions may be very useful in developing organ-donation campaigns based on psychological persuasion techniques (Alcalay, 1983; Flay, 1985, 1987; Maccoby & Farquhar, 1977; Maccoby & Solomon, 1981). In addition, insights gained from studies of individual differences in attitudes about organ donation may help in formulating campaigns targeting particular populations.

RATIONALE FOR THE CONFERENCE AND BOOK

When we first began considering organizing the conference, there were, to our knowledge, about two dozen behavioral investigators conducting research on psychological aspects of organ donation.[1] As discussed previously, these investigators were scattered in a variety of areas, departments, and disciplines. Too often, these diverse scholars were unaware of each other's efforts. The consequences of this lack of interaction were redundancies and uncoordinated research efforts. In addition, the results of the various efforts had not been effectively disseminated due to the scattering of relevant articles across journals in so many areas.

There was a need to bring these researchers together to allow communication in formal and informal settings. One way to remedy the problem was to have a conference of investigators interested in organ donation.

Conference Plan

The conference was a two-day meeting of 25 psychologists and other behavioral scientists involved in research on organ donation. In addition, several transplant coordinators and educators attended the conference. Funding was provided by the American Psychological Association, the Division of Organ Transplantation of the Public Health Service, U.S. Department of Health and Human Services, and Kansas State University.

On the first day of the conference, there were two keynote presentations by Jeffrey Prottas and Roger Evans. Following these addresses, the other research participants gave brief presentations of their specific research programs and conceptual approaches. Each of the sessions of 5–6 papers concluded with a brief discussion by a noted research psychologist not intimately involved in organ donation research. The first day concluded with a banquet and address by Jane Warmbrodt, Professional Education Specialist with Sandoz Pharmaceuticals Corporation.

---

1. We have since become aware of over a dozen more psychologists who have worked on issues related to organ donation and transplantation.

The second day began with some comments from the transplant coordinators and educators to the previous day's presentations. They reacted to the specific presentations, but, more important, they sketched an overview research framework to be used in planning future behavioral research on organ donation. Edi Servino, director of the United Network on Organ Sharing, coordinated this effort. The conference concluded in the afternoon with tentative planning for a second conference on the topic and a discussion of future plans for coordinating communication by electronic mail.[2]

Throughout the conference, informal interaction among the participants was encouraged. As most of the invitees had not previously met each other, such interaction was vital to breaking down personal and professional barriers among researchers.

ORGANIZATION OF THE BOOK

The rest of this book is organized into four parts. The first two parts present results from empirical research on psychological aspects of organ donation. Some of the studies used laboratory research on individual subjects, others involved survey research, and still others used field studies of families who have faced the organ donation decision. The first part includes the studies with an individual perspective, and the second part includes those taking a group perspective. The third part is more conceptual than empirical and deals with possible policy implications, social marketing strategies, and connections to other areas of study. Finally, the fourth part presents three responses adapted from the remarks presented by the discussants and a brief conclusion by the editors. None of the three discussants had themselves conducted research in organ donation, but rather have expertise in consumer decision making and living wills (Lola Lopes), social psychology and social cognition (David Schneider), or public policy research (Kenneth Hammond). They bring an "outside" perspective in response to the research.

The backgrounds of the major contributors are difficult to categorize neatly, as several are currently working in areas other than that of their formal training. The group consists of cognitive psychologists (Shanteau, Harris, and Nolan), social psychologists (Skowronski, Borgida, Lefcourt, Hessing, Piliavin, and Shepherd), a clinical psychologist (Perkins), sociologists (Simmons and Batten), marketing researchers (Belk, Thukral, Johnson, and Fox), and students (Jasper, Smith, and Linin).

Organizing the conference and this book has been an intellectually exciting endeavor for us. We hope that the readers will catch a little of that excitement from reading these chapters.

---

2. There is now a network established with a bulletin board and literature list available by BITNET (contact JSHANTEAU @ KSUVM or RJHARRIS @ KSUVM).

References

Alcalay, R. (1983). The impact of mass communication campaigns in the health field. *Social Science and Medicine, 17*, 87–94.

Andersen, K. S., & Fox, D. M. (1988). The impact of routine inquiry laws on organ donation. *Health Affairs, 7*(5), 65–78.

Anderson, B. F., Deane, D. H., Hammond, K. R., McClelland, G. H., & Shanteau, J. C. (1981). *Concepts in judgment and decision research: Definitions, sources, inter-relations, comments.* New York: Praeger.

Baldwin, D. (1987, May/June). Politics to the rescue. *Common Cause Magazine,* p. 7.

Barach, J. A. (1984, July/August). Applying marketing princicples to social causes. *Business Horizons,* pp. 65–69.

Barnett, M. A. (1987). Empathy and related responses in children. In N. Eisenberg & J. Strayer (Eds.), *Empathy and its development* (pp. 146–162) New York: Cambridge University Press.

Barnett, M. A., Klassen, M. L., McMinimy, V., & Schwarz, L. (1987). The role of self- and other-oriented motivation in the organ donation decision. *Advances in Consumer Research, 14,* 335–337.

Bart, K. J., Macon, E. J., Humphries, A. L., Baldwin, R. J., Fitch, T., Pope, R. S., Rich, M. J., Langford, D., Teutsch, S. M., & Blount, J. H. (1981). Increasing the supply of cadaveric kidneys for transplantation. *Transplantation, 31,* 383–387.

Belk, R. W., & Austin, M. C. (1986). Organ donation willingness as a function of extended self and materialism. In M. Venkatesen (Ed.), *Advances in Health Care Research.* Snowbird, UT: Association for Health Care Research.

Bloom, P. N., & Novelli, W. D. (1981). Problems and challenges in social marketing. *Journal of Marketing, 45*(2), 79–88.

Callender, C. O. (1987). Organ donation in the black population: Where to go from here? *Transplantation Proceedings, 19* (Suppl. 2), 36–40.

Caplan, A. (1984). Ethical and policy issues in the procurement of cadaver organs for transplantation. *New England Journal of Medicine, 311*(15), 981–983.

Clark, M., Robinson, C., & Wickelgren, I. (1988, September 12). Interchangeable parts. *Newsweek,* pp. 61, 63.

Cleveland, S. (1975). Changes in human tissue donor attitudes: 1969–1974. *Psychosomatic Medicine, 37*(4), 306–312.

Corlett, S. (1985). Public attitudes toward human organ donation. *Transplantation Proceedings, 17*(Suppl. 3), 103–110.

Eisenberg, N. (1982). *The development of prosocial behavior.* New York: Academic Press.

Evans, R., & Manninen, D. (1988, October). U.S. public opinion concerning the procurement and distribution of donor organs. *Transplantation Proceedings, 20*(5), 781–785.

Evans, R., Manninen, D., Gersh, B., Hart, G., & Rodin, J. (1984). The need for and supply of donor hearts for transplantation. *Journal of Heart Transplantations, 4*(1), 57–60.

Fellner, C. H., & Marshall, J. R. (1981). Kidney donors revisited. In J. P. Rushton & R. M. Sorrentino (Eds.), *Altruism and helping behavior* (pp.351–365). Hillsdale, NJ: Erlbaum.

Flay, B. R. (1985). Psychosocial approaches to smoking prevention: A review of findings. *Health Psychology, 4,* 449–488.

Flay, B. R. (1987). Mass media and smoking cessation: A critical review. *American Journal of Public Health, 77*(2), 153–160.

Fox, K., & Kotler, P. (1980). The marketing of social causes: The first 10 years. *Journal of Marketing, 44*(4), 24–33.

Francisco, C. J. (1987). Legislature adds new life to organ donation, transplantation. *Texas Medicine, 83*(10), 55–58.

Frauman, A. C., & Miles, M. S. (1987). Parental willingness to donate the organs of a child. *ANNA Journal, 14*(6), 401–404.

Fulton, J., Fulton, R., & Simmons, R. G. (1977). The cadaver organ and the gift of life. In R. G. Simmons, S. Klein, and R. L. Simmons (Eds.), *Gift of life: The social and psychological impact of organ transplantation* (pp. 338–376). New York: Wiley.

Greenfield, J. (1988). The media and the transplant issue: Why they do what they do. *Transplantation Proceedings, 20* (1, Suppl. 1), 1038–1040.

Gunby, P. (1983). Media-abetted liver transplants raise questions of "equity and decency." *Journal of the American Medical Association, 249*(15), 1973–1982.

Guy, B. S., & Patton, W. E. (1989). The marketing of altruistic causes: Understanding why people help. *Journal of Consumer Marketing, 6*(1), 19–30.

Haney, C. A. (1973). Issues and considerations in requesting an anatomical gift. *Social Science and Medicine, 7*, 635–642.

Hessing, D. J., & Elffers, H. (1986). Attitude toward death, fear of being declared dead too soon, and donation of organs after death. *Omega, 17*, 115–126.

Hosten, A. O. (1987). Kidney disease in Blacks in North America: An overview. *Transplantation Proceedings*, 19 (Suppl. 2), 5–8.

Hostetler, A. J. (1987, August). Transplants boast long history, recent success. *APA Monitor*, p. 24.

Johnson, L., Lum, C., Thompson, T., Wilson, J., Urdaneta, M., & Harris, R. (1988). Mexican-American and Anglo-American attitudes toward organ donation. *Transplantation Proceedings, 20*(5), 822–823.

Jones, D. B. (1988). A second chance. *Texas Medicine, 84*(12), 86–88.

Kalter, J. (1986, August 30). Is TV helping the neediest—or the cutest? *TV Guide.*

Krasner, W. L., & Bailey, W. A. (1986). Grants policy implementation: When the media loses interest. *Grants Magazine, 9*(2), pp. 80–84.

Maccoby, N., & Farquhar, J. W. (1977). Reducing the risk of cardiovascular disease: Effects of a community-based campaign on knowledge and behavior. *Journal of Community Health, 3*(2).

Maccoby, N., & Solomon, D. S. (1981). The Stanford community studies in heart disease prevention. In R. Rice and W. Paisley (Eds.), *Public communication campaigns*. Beverly Hills: Sage.

Manninen, D., & Evans, R. (1985). Public attitudes and behavior regarding organ donation. *Journal of the American Medical Association, 253*(21), 3111–3115.

Manning, P., & McCabe, R. (1986). Limiting factors in the gift of life. In M. A. Hardy, M. L. Orr, C. S. Torres, & L. Parsonnet (Eds.), *Positive approaches to living with end-stage renal disease* (pp. 32–36). New York: Praeger.

Martyn, S., Wright, R., & Clark, L. (1988, April/May). Required request for organ donation: Moral, clinical, and legal problems. *The Hastings Center Report, 18*, 27–34.

McIntyre, P., Barnett, M. A., Harris, R. J., Shanteau, J., Skowronski, J. J., & Klassen, M. (1987). Psychological factors influencing decisions to donate organs. *Advances in Consumer Research, 14*, 331–334.

Moores, B., Clarke, G., Lewis, B. R., & Mallick, N. P. (1976). Public attitudes toward kidney transplantation. *British Medical Journal, 1*, 629–631.

Nuckolls, E. (1989, October). *Identifying organ donor family needs.* Paper presented at Tulane Symposium on Organ Donation, New Orleans, LA.

Olbrisch, M. E. (1989). Psychology's contribution to relieving the donor organ shortage: Barriers from within. *American Psychologist, 44*(1), 77–78.

Parisi, V., & Katz, I. (1986). Attitudes toward posthumous organ donation and commitment to donate. *Health Psychology, 5*(6), 565–580.

Perkins, K. (1987). The shortage of cadaver donor organs for transplantation: Can psychology help? *American Psychologist, 42*(10), 921–930.

Perez, L., Matas, A., & Tellis, U. (1988). Organ donation in three major U.S. cities by race/ethnicity. *Transplantation Proceedings, 20*, 815.

Pessemier, E. A., Bemmaor, A. C., & Hanssens, D. M. (1977). Willingness to supply human body parts: Some empirical results. *Journal of Consumer Research, 4*, 131–140.

Pollak, R., Prusak, B. F., Wiberg, C. A., & Mozes, M. F. (1986). Donor referral and organ procurement patterns in a large metropolitan area—a single center prospective study. *Transplantation Proceedings, 18,* 399–400.

Prottas, J. (1983). Encouraging altruism: Public attitudes and the marketing of organ donation. *Milbank Memorial Fund Quarterly/Health and Society, 61*(2), 278–306.

Rothschild, M. L. (1979). Marketing communications in nonbusiness situations or why it's so hard to sell brotherhood like soap. *Journal of Marketing, 43*(2), 11–20.

Royster, B., Tetreault, P., & Shanteau, J. (1987, May). *Death anxiety, social desirability, and gender differences: Influences on organ donation.* Paper presented at the meeting of the Midwestern Psychological Association, Chicago, IL.

Rushton, J. P., & Sorrentino, R. M. (1981). *Altruism and helping behavior: Social, personality, and developmental perspectives.* Hillsdale, NJ: Erlbaum.

Shanteau, J. (1986). Psychological research on organ donation. In M. Venkatesan (Ed.), *Proceedings of the fifth annual health care conference.* Snowbird, UT: Association for Health Care Research.

Sipes, D. D. (1987). State, federal statutes guide organ donation procedures. *Health Progress, 68*(5), 46–50, 67.

Skowronski, J. J. (1987, May). *Psychological factors influencing decisions to donate organs.* Paper presented at the meeting of the Midwestern Psychological Association, Chicago, IL.

Sojka, J. R. Z. (1985). Understanding donor behavior: A classification paradigm. *Advances in Consumer Research, 13,* 240–245.

Thukral, V. K., & Cummins, G. (1987). The vital organ shortage. *Advances in Nonprofit Marketing, 2,* 159–174.

U.S. Department of Health and Human Services (1986, September 30). Press release issued by Public Health Service.

U.S. Department of Health and Human Services (1988, January 28). Press release issued by Public Health Service.

Warmbrodt, J., & Koch, C. (1985). *National organ transplantation facts.* Kansas City, MO: Midwest Organ Bank.

Weedn, V. M., & Leveque, B. (1988). Routine inquiry for organ and tissue donations. *Texas Medicine, 84*(12), 30–37.

Wilms, G., Kiefer, S. W., Shanteau, J., & McIntyre, P. (1987). Knowledge and image of body organs: Impact on willingness to donate. *Advances in Consumer Research, 14,* 338–341.

Winkel, F. W. (1984). Public communication on donor cards: A comparison of persuasive styles. *Social Science and Medicine, 19,* 957–963.

Youngner, S. J., Allen, M., Bartlett, E. T., Cascorbi, H. F., Hau, T., Jackson, D. L., Mahowald, M. B., & Martin, B. J. (1985). Psychosocial and ethical implications of organ retrieval. *New England Journal of Medicine, 313,* 321–324.

PART ONE

INDIVIDUAL AND COGNITIVE FACTORS

CHAPTER 2

ORGAN DONATION CONSENT DECISIONS BY THE NEXT OF KIN:
AN EXPERIMENTAL SIMULATION APPROACH

RICHARD JACKSON HARRIS, JOHN DAVID JASPER,
JAMES SHANTEAU, STACY A. SMITH

Regardless of whether or not a donor card is signed, the final decision about organ donation is usually made by the donor's family after his or her death (Childress, 1987; Lee & Kissner, 1986; Overcast, Evans, Bowen, Hoe, & Livak, 1984; Peters, 1986; Prottas, 1985; Schwindt & Vining, 1986; Somerville, 1985). The decision to donate the organs of a next of kin may be seen as a cognitive issue affected by the way information is sought, evaluated, and combined. One of the keys to understanding the psychology of organ donation, therefore, is to analyze what factors influence the decision and to determine how these factors are integrated.

The extreme emotional stress surrounding the decision to donate the organs of a next of kin makes it very difficult to study the decision-making process. Nonetheless, some field and observational studies have identified several important factors affecting the decision, such as the presence of supportive others, allowing the survivors time to absorb the shock of the death, and the sensitivity of the approach to the family (Bart et al., 1981; Fulton, Fulton, & Simmons, 1977; Haney, 1973; Manning & McCabe, 1986). The most effective appeals are those that provide needed information in a sensitive and tactful manner, as well as refute misconceptions about organ donation (Parisi & Katz, 1986; Winkel, 1984; Youngner et al., 1985).

The study discussed in this chapter focused on the information that people use in making a decision about donating the organs of a recently deceased next of kin. In an experimental simulation approach, subjects read brief scenarios describing a situation in which a decision must be made by some hypothetical next of kin. Each story ended with a question about whether consent to donate should be given; the subjects were asked to answer "yes," "no," or "undecided" and to write their reasons for their choices. Every story had two versions; each subject received only one of the two versions. The versions were identical except for a slight change of wording regarding one critical issue that previous research had suggested as being important. Thus, results indicated whether the change of information made a difference in responses. A brief attitude survey about organ donation was also taken, and results were correlated with responses on the decision task.

METHOD

Materials

Fifteen brief scenarios of 55 to 130 words were written. Each described a young adult who had recently died a sudden and untimely death and whose kin were now facing the decision of whether or not to donate their loved one's organs. Each scenario had two versions, identical except for a wording change regarding a critical issue. In the examples that follow this section, italicized portions varied across the two versions in each story. These portions were not italicized in what the subjects read. The issues examined were (a) signing or not signing a donor card, (b) heart death versus brain death, (c) decedent's attitude toward organ donation, (d) abortion versus miscarriage for a fetal donor, (e) attitudes of next of kin, (f) intended use of organs, (g) particular organs donated, (h) decedent's attitude toward doctors, (i) decedent's religious beliefs, (j) decedent's character, (k) wording of the consent form, (l) age of decedent, (m) manner of death, (n) type of funeral, and (o) decedent's belief about bodily resurrection. Several sample stories in both versions follow:

Story 1A: Barry Johnson
Barry Johnson, a freshman at Kansas State University (KSU), has just been killed in a tragic motorcycle accident after his cycle ran off the highway and into a bridge abutment. His body is now lying in the hospital while the organ transplant coordinator is talking with Barry's distraught parents about the possibility of donating his organs. As his parents consider this request to give permission to take Barry's organs, they see that *he had signed the back of his driver's license indicating his wish to have his organs donated upon his death.* The transplant coordinator carefully explains that their permission is necessary before the organs may be used. Should Barry's parents consent to have his organs donated?

Story 1B: Barry Johnson
Barry Johnson, a freshman at KSU, has just been killed in a tragic motorcycle accident after his cycle ran off the highway and into a bridge abutment.

His body is now lying in the hospital while the organ transplant coordinator is talking with Barry's distraught parents about the possibility of donating his organs. As his parents consider this request to give permission to take Barry's organs, they see that *he had not signed the back of his driver's license. Thus they had no idea what their son's wishes about organ donation had been.* The transplant coordinator carefully explains that their permission is necessary before the organs may be used. Should Barry's parents consent to have his organs donated?

Story 10A: Rob Williams
After attending his high school graduation party, Rob Williams was killed in a terrible car accident on his way home. Rob was known at school as *a loner and a troublemaker.* Rob *never* seemed interested in the problems and concerns of other students. He was the kind of person who *always* got into trouble. Should Rob's parents consent to have his organs donated?

Story 10B: Rob Williams
After attending his high school graduation party, Rob Williams was killed in a terrible car accident on his way home. Rob was known at school *as a very popular student.* Rob *always* seemed interested in the problems and concerns of other students. He was the kind of person who *never* got into trouble. Should Rob's parents consent to have his organs donated?

Procedure

The subjects were 295 introductory psychology students who participated as part of a course requirement. They were recruited for a study of the "Evaluation of Moral Dilemmas." No mention of organ donation was made on the sign-up sheet, in order to avoid self-selection biases. Both the subjects and the characters in the stories were 18 to 25 years of age, which is the optimal age for organs to be donated. Subjects were tested in groups of 15–25 per session.

The subjects were told, "This experiment is part of an ongoing project on psychological aspects of organ donation. We are looking at such issues as why people would agree or not agree to become an organ donor themselves or consent to donate someone else's organs upon the person's death. This particular experiment today asks you to read several brief scenarios of hypothetical people in hypothetical situations where they face a moral dilemma and must make a choice about organ donation."

Subjects were asked to indicate whether they thought the surviving relatives should or should not agree to donate the organs of the deceased or whether they were uncertain what that person should do. They were then asked to write down their reasons for their choices and were told, "There are no right or wrong answers; we are only interested in how people approach these situations. Though we realize this may not be a pleasant topic to think about, we hope that the time spent on it in this experiment will help clarify your own knowledge and thinking about this very serious and increasingly important moral and medical issue." The subjects were instructed to work at their own speed and to ask any questions that they had.

The students first completed a demographic questionnaire, which gathered information on gender, ethnic background, education, college major, religion, and marital status, as well as information about their present attitude on organ donation. Specifically, they were asked to check one of the following options about whether they had signed a donor card: "yes"; "no, but I'd be willing to do so if asked"; "no, but I might consider doing so in the future"; "no, I thought about it and decided not to"; or "no, I didn't even know about it."

The 15 stories were presented on sheets of paper, with three to four stories per page. To partially counterbalance the presentation sequence of the stories, subjects passed the four pages around the group and answered the questions for each page of stories on a separate answer sheet. Thus each set of three to four stories was read first, second, third, or fourth by approximately one fourth of the subjects. For each story, subjects checked "yes," "no," or "I'm undecided" and then gave reasons for their decisions. Subjects worked at their own speed. The session lasted 45–50 minutes.

RESULTS

Demographics

Overall the sample was gender-balanced (48% men, 52% women), predominately White (92%), never married (96%), freshman (74%), and Christian (82%). Almost everyone (97.3%) had heard about organ donation, with friends and the media reported most often as sources of that information. Whereas only 9% had signed a donor card (donors), 23% said they would be willing to do so if asked (willings), and another 54% said that they might consider doing so in the future (undecideds). Only 12% indicated that they had decided not to sign a donor card (nondonors); 2% reported not knowing about the donor card on the back of their driver's licenses (uninformed). This is consistent with past research (e.g., McIntyre et al., 1987; see also chapter 11, by J. J. Skowronski in this volume) and suggests that a large number of people who have as yet made no commitment to become organ donors may very likely agree to it with some persuasion, and perhaps with only a request.

The relations of gender and of religious preference to willingness to donate appear in Table 1. There were no differences in the numbers of men and women in the donor or undecided categories, but there were somewhat more women than men in the willing category, whereas the reverse was true for the nondonors.

In terms of religion, there were few differences across the various Christian categories, except for somewhat fewer donors among Catholics and slightly fewer nondonors among "born-again" Christians. Among those indicating no religion, however, a different pattern emerged. Whereas there were only about half as many undecideds as there were in the three Christian groups, both the number of willings and nondonors was considerably larger than the other groups. It seems that those indicating no religion are less undecided than the Christians, although

Table 1

DISTRIBUTION OF SUBJECTS BY RELIGION AND GENDER ACROSS DONOR
CATEGORIES (%)

Category	No religious preference	Catholic	Protestant	"Born-again" Christian	Men	Women	Overall
Donors	10.2	4.5	11.6	10.3	8.5	9.8	9.2
Willings	34.7	19.1	20.7	24.1	18.3	26.8	22.7
Undecideds	30.6	62.9	55.4	58.6	53.5	54.2	53.9
Nondonors	20.4	12.4	10.7	6.9	16.2	9.2	12.5
Uninformed	4.1	1.1	1.7	0.0	3.5	0.0	1.7
n	49	89	121	29	142	153	295

Note. Column totals may not equal 100% due to rounding error.

the decisions divided into for and against proportionately to the rest of the population.

Decision Data

The frequencies of yes, no, and undecided responses were tabulated for each story in each condition. These results appear in Table 2. Considering the group data, some consistent trends were apparent. Results are reported with 95 percent confidence intervals around the means in parentheses in the text. Only data from the stories discussed herein and that showed significant differences appear in the table.

Wishes of the Deceased

A conclusion drawn from the responses for several of the stories is that the most important variable in the responses seemed to be the wishes of the deceased. For example, in Story 3, 94% (±3.8) of the subjects said that the wife should donate her husband's organs if he had strong feelings in favor of organ donation, and 86% (±5.6) said she should not donate if he had strong feelings against. In Story 1, 98% (±2.3) said surviving parents should donate the organs of a son who had signed a donor card. When he had not signed the card and thus his feelings were unknown, only 39% (±7.8) recommended donating, and 37% (±7.8) were undecided. The preferences of the survivors, on the other hand, had only a modest effect (Story 5). When the victim had signed a donor card and the next of kin also supported donation, 99% (±1.6) recommended donation. When the next of kin were against donation in the same instance, the percentage recommending donation dropped only to 87% (±5.4).

More indirect indications of the importance of the victim's preference can be seen in the responses to Stories 8 and 15. In Story 15, when the victim believed that only her spirit or soul would rise to heaven, 86% (±5.6) decided to

Table 2

DONOR DECISIONS (%) BY STORY VERSION AND SUBJECT DONOR TYPE

	n	Yes %	No %	Undecided %
Story 1				
A Donor signed donor card		**98**	1	1
Donor or willing subjects	54	98	0	0
Undecided subjects	77	99	0	1
Nondonor subjects	15	93	7	0
B Donor did not sign card		**39**	**24**	**37**
Donor or willing subjects	40	62	12	25
Undecided subjects	82	33	20	48
Nondonor subjects	22	14	68	18
Story 3				
A Strong donor feelings for		**94**	3	2
Donor or willing subjects	54	96	2	0
Undecided subjects	77	96	0	4
Nondonor subjects	15	73	27	0
B Strong donor feelings against		**8**	**86**	6
Donor or willing subjects	40	18	72	10
Undecided subjects	82	2	92	6
Nondonor subjects	22	9	91	0
Story 5				
A Strong kin feelings for		**99**	0	1
Donor or willing subjects	54	100	0	0
Undecided subjects	77	99	0	1
Nondonor subjects	15	100	0	0
B Strong kin feelings against		**87**	5	7
Donor or willing subjects	40	90	0	10
Undecided subjects	82	87	7	6
Nondonor subjects	22	86	4	9
Story 6				
A Organs for research		**42**	16	42
Donor or willing subjects	54	56	7	41
Undecided subjects	77	38	13	49
Nondonor subjects	15	27	60	13
B Organs for transplantation		**76**	3	**20**
Donor or willing subjects	40	85	0	15
Undecided subjects	82	77	5	18
Nondonor subjects	22	64	4	32
Story 8				
A Donor distrusted doctors		**19**	**58**	22
Donor or willing subjects	54	24	54	22
Undecided subjects	77	17	57	25
Nondonor subjects	15	13	80	7
B Donor admired doctors		**90**	1	**10**
Donor or willing subjects	40	93	0	8
Undecided subjects	82	88	1	11
Nondonor subjects	22	91	0	9

Table 2, continued

	n	Yes %	No %	Undecided %
Story 10				
A Donor a loner and a troublemaker		**55**	**17**	**28**
Donor or willing subjects	54	67	6	28
Undecided subjects	77	54	18	27
Nondonor subjects	15	20	53	27
B Donor concerned and caring		**90**	**1**	**9**
Donor or willing subjects	40	95	0	5
Undecided subjects	82	88	1	10
Nondonor subjects	22	91	0	9
Story 14				
A Open-casket funeral		**39**	**31**	**31**
Donor or willing subjects	54	54	26	20
Undecided subjects	77	32	27	40
Nondonor subjects	15	20	60	20
B Cremation		**47**	**30**	**22**
Donor or willing subjects	40	65	10	25
Undecided subjects	82	45	32	23
Nondonor subjects	22	27	54	18
Story 15				
A Donor believed only soul rises		**86**	**5**	**9**
Donor or willing subjects	54	96	4	0
Undecided subjects	77	83	3	14
Nondonor subjects	15	60	27	13
B Donor believed soul and body rise		**16**	**60**	**24**
Donor or willing subjects	40	25	35	40
Undecided subjects	82	12	70	18
Nondonor subjects	22	9	68	23

Note. Percentages may not total 100 due to rounding error.

donate; when she believed that her physical body would rise as well, 60% ($\pm$7.9) decided not to donate. This seems to reflect an inference of and a respect for the victim's wishes. In Story 8, 90% ($\pm$4.8) approved of donating the organs of a woman said to trust and respect doctors, whereas only 19% ($\pm$6.3) chose to donate if the deceased had mistrusted and disliked doctors. Even this more indirect indication affected the donation decision.

Character Contamination

A few other variables affected the donation decisions. One was that subjects seemed to value the organs of someone whose character they deemed more worthy than someone they deemed less worthy. This applied even in cases where there could be no plausible effect on the quality of the organs. For example, in Story 10, subjects were more likely to recommend donation of the organs of an upstanding, caring young man (90%, ±4.8) than a loner and a troublemaker (55%, ±8.0).

This finding of "contamination" of the organs of the victim by his or her character is an interesting one, and the contamination was also seen in other ways. Although the religion of the deceased (Story 9) would seem to be one of those nondiagnostic factors in the subjects' decisions, a closer look suggested otherwise. In a breakdown of Story 9 by subjects' religious preferences (see Table 3), people were more likely to recommend donating the organs of someone of similar religious beliefs. Christians are more likely to donate the organs of another Christian (Story 9A), whereas no-religion subjects are more likely to donate the organs of an atheist (Story 9B). Unfortunately, the low total sample number in some of the cells led to wider confidence intervals than needed for statistical significance. This character contamination issue had not been expected or previously discovered and requires further study.

Other Bases of Decisions

Subjects also were significantly more likely to advocate donating organs for use in transplantation (76%, ±6.9) than for use in research (42%, ±8.0; Story 6). They were slightly more likely to approve of donation if cremation (47%, ±8.0), rather than an open-casket funeral (39%, ±7.9), were planned (Story 14).

The crucial variables in several of the other stories had no effect on the decisions to donate. It made no difference whether the specifications were "heart death" or "brain death" (Story 2), fetal tissue from an abortion or miscarriage (Story 4), heart–lung or cornea transplant (Story 7), wording of the consent form

Table 3

DONATION DECISIONS FOR STORY 9 BY SUBJECT RELIGIOUS PREFERENCE (%)

		Yes	No	Undecided
Story 9	n	%	%	%
A (Donor a fundamentalist)		65 (±7.7)	11 (±5.0)	24 (±6.9)
Subject's religion				
No religion	17	47 (±23.7)	24 (±20.3)	29 (±21.6)
Catholic	44	61 (±14.4)	5 (±6.4)	34 (±14.0)
Protestant	67	70 (±11.0)	12 (±7.8)	16 (±8.8)
"Born-again" Christian	15	80 (±20.2)	0	20 (±20.2)
B (Donor an atheist)		60 (±7.9)	14 (±5.6)	26 (±7.1)
Subject's religion				
No religion	32	72 (±15.6)	13 (±11.6)	16 (±12.7)
Catholic	45	60 (±14.3)	11 (±9.1)	29 (±13.2)
Protestant	54	57 (±13.2)	19 (±10.5)	24 (±11.4)
"Born-again" Christian	14	50 (±26.2)	7 (±13.4)	43 (±25.9)

Note. Ninety-five percent confidence intervals are in parentheses.

(Story 11), age of the deceased (Story 12), or suicide versus accidental death (Story 13).

There are two possible reasons for the "no effect" results: (a) Subjects considered the key variables, but decided they were unimportant, or (b) subjects never looked at the key variables (see discussion of reasons in following section).

Examination by Subject Donor Category

Based on their responses to the demographic questionnaire described previously, subjects were divided into donors, willings, undecideds, nondonors, and the uninformed. Donor decisions were tallied separately for each group. These data are presented also in Table 2, with the donor and willing groups' percentages combined, due to the relatively small numbers in the donor category. The uninformed subjects' data are not presented, since they constituted less than 2 percent of the entire sample. Generally, the more favorably disposed toward organ donation the subject was, the more likely he or she was to suggest donation for the character in the story. However, as can be seen from the table, information in the story was far more influential a factor than the subject's own attitude. For example, in the responses to several stories (e.g., Stories 1A, 3A, 5A, 5B, 8B, and 10B) even nondonors overwhelmingly recommended donation (see chapter 3 by B. E. Noland and P. J. McGrath, and chapter 6, by J. Shanteau and J. J. Skowronski in this volume). In the responses to others, however—Stories 3B, 8A, and 15B—confirmed donors recommended against donation. This suggests that, although influenced by their own attitudes, subjects on both ends of the opinion spectrum based their decisions largely on their understanding of the wishes of the deceased person.

Reasons for Decisions

Scoring of Reasons

Reasons given for the responses were scored according to the following scale:

1. Direct   Subject acknowledged the target information by mentioning the target information or its perceived meaning literally.
2. Indirect   Subject mentioned the target information, but obliquely or indirectly, citing either a related issue or alluding to the results of such an issue.
3. Other   Subject gave other reason(s) completely unrelated to the target information.
4. No Response   Subject left the space for writing reasons blank.

The responses were scored by two of the authors (Jasper and Smith) with consultation with a third (Harris) for questionable cases.

Results

Frequencies of the different classes of reasons were calculated. Two aspects of the reasons data are noteworthy. First, in many of the stories, more than 90% of the subjects mentioned a direct or indirect reason (Stories 1A, 3A, 3B, 14B, and 15B). For others, more than 90% did not (11A, 11B, 12A, and 13B). The latter may be because subjects did not see that information as important (e.g., wording of the donation consent form) or did not see it as distinctive (e.g., victim was a young adult or an accident victim); in the latter cases, many subjects commented on the version with the less typical information (e.g., victim a child or suicide victim).

A second aspect of the data on reasons given for decisions may be seen in the breakdown of reasons for donation choice. For Story 1B, for example, subjects who mentioned the key information that the victim had not signed his donor card were much more likely to recommend not donating than subjects who did not mention that information (34% vs. 4%). A parallel result was seen in Story 8A, where 68% of subjects mentioning the victim's distrust of doctors recommended not donating, while only 31% of subjects not mentioning that information did so. Finally, for Story 15, subjects who mentioned the relevant theological information overwhelmingly recommended donating (95%) if the donor believed that only the soul rose (story version 15A), and against donating (67%) if the donor believed both the body and soul rose (15B). Subjects not identifying the religious belief as a factor in their decision showed responses more evenly scattered across the response categories.

In conclusion, examination of the reasons mentioned confirmed that subjects were making their decisions for many of the stories based on the variables deemed by the experimenters to be relevant. The results, however, varied widely across the stories. Generally, subjects not mentioning these reasons showed closer to a random distribution of responses across the three response categories.

DISCUSSION

This study has demonstrated the productive use of an experimental simulation methodology to examine the psychology of decisions about organ donation. The scenario technique yielded some readily interpretable results of a sort not readily obtainable from survey methodology. The most important influence on the donation decision is the subject's perception of the wishes of the deceased about organ donation. Such wishes may have been indicated overtly, such as a direct statement or the signing of a donor card, or more indirectly in ways such as a general attitude toward doctors. A second strong finding involved the character contamination effect, whereby subjects are more likely to donate the organs of a person of positive character or similar attitudes and values to their own. This methodology has applicability to studying the role of still more variables in the decision process. For example, Jasper, Harris, Lee, and Miller (1989) examined the effect of offering the next of kin explanations about such terms as "brain death."

There are, of course, some limitations with this methodology. First, the subjects are asked to recommend a decision for someone else, which may be very different than what they would in fact choose themselves. In some sense, the subject is inferring what the next of kin would have inferred about the wishes of the victim. Second, the extreme stress and emotional trauma in a real donation situation is, of course, not reproducible in the laboratory (see chapter 18, by L. Lopes in this volume). Nevertheless, in defense of this methodology, the two versions of each story are identical except for the critical target information. Thus any differences in decisions must be attributable to that variable. The ultimate value of this methodology may be to identify issues for study in a more natural-istic context.

Although this study examined several possible bases for making a donation decision for a next of kin, one issue not explored is how the various pieces of information might interact. Subjects were given one scenario in which the vic-tim's signing a donor card was the variable, another with the attitudes of the next of kin as the variable, and so forth. However, the possible interaction of multiple pieces of target information within the same story was not investigated. Research by Harris, Jasper, Lee, and Miller (1989) varied two pieces of information orthogonally within a story and strongly confirmed the dominant role of the perceived wishes of the deceased. Subjects consistently weighted the potential donor's attitude far more heavily than their own attitudes or those of the donor's next of kin.

Some implications for organ donation policy may be drawn from the present study. A next of kin appears far more likely to consent to donation if he or she believes that the deceased would want to donate. Given the generally positive attitude toward donation expressed by our students, encouraging more people to discuss the issues with their families would help ensure that positive feelings about organ donation are known by family members.

Although a signed donor card is not considered sufficient for a transplant team to remove an organ, it can still be a vital intermediate step in obtaining consent from the next of kin. If the next of kin rely heavily even on indirect indicators like theology or trust in doctors, then how much more helpful would they find a clear and unequivocal statement of the deceased's wishes! A signed donor card provides just such a statement. The next of kin can then take some comfort in being certain that their consent to donate reflected the true wishes of their loved one.

References

Bart, K. J., Macon, E. J., Humphries, A. L., Baldwin, R. J., Fitch, T., Pope, R. S., Rich, M. J., Langford, D., Teutsch, S. M., & Blount, J. H. (1981). Increasing the supply of cadaveric kidneys for transplantation. *Transplantation, 31*, 383–387.
Childress, J. F. (1987). Some moral connections between organ procurement and organ distribution. *Journal of Contemporary Health Law and Policy, 3*, 85–110.

Fulton, J., Fulton, R., & Simmons, R. G. (1977). The cadaver organ and the gift of life. In R. G. Simmons, S. Klein, and R. L. Simmons (Eds.), *Gift of life: The social and psychological impact of organ transplantation* (pp. 338-376). New York: Wiley.

Haney, C. A. (1973). Issues and considerations in requesting an anatomical gift. *Social Science and Medicine, 7,* 635-642.

Harris, R. J., Jasper, J. D., Lee, B. C., & Miller, K. E. (1989). *Consenting to donate organs: Whose wishes carry the most weight?* Manuscript submitted for publication.

Jasper, J. D., Harris, R. J., Lee, B. C., & Miller, K. E. (1989). *Organ donation terminology: Are we communicating life or death?* Manuscript submitted for publication.

Lee, P. P., & Kissner, P. (1986). Organ donation and the Uniform Anatomical Gift Act. *Surgery, 100* (5), 867-875.

Manning, P., & McCabe, R. (1986). Limiting factors in the gift of life. In M. A. Hardy, M. L. Orr, C. S. Torres, & L. Parsonnet (Eds.), *Positive approaches to living with end-stage renal disease* (pp. 32-36). New York: Praeger.

McIntyre, P., Barnett, M. A., Harris, R. J., Shanteau, J., Skowronski, J. J., & Klassen, M. (1987). Psychological factors influencing decision to donate organs. *Advances in Consumer Research, 14,* 331-334.

Overcast, T. D., Evans, R. W., Bowen, L. E., Hoe, M. M., & Livak, C. L. (1984). Problems in the identification of potential organ donors: Misconceptions and fallacies associated with donor cards. *Journal of the American Medical Association, 251*(22), 1559-1562.

Parisi, V., & Katz, I. (1986). Attitudes toward posthumous organ donation and commitment to donate. *Health Psychology, 5,* 565-580.

Peters, D. A. (1986). Protecting autonomy in organ procurement procedures: Some overlooked issues. *Milbank Memorial Fund Quarterly, 64*(2), 241-270.

Prottas, J. M. (1985). Organ procurement in Europe and the United States. *Milbank Memorial Fund Quarterly, 63*(1), 94-126.

Schwindt, R., & Vining, A. R. (1986). Proposal for a future delivery market for transplanted organs. *Journal of Health Politics, Policy and Law, 11*(3), 483-500.

Somerville, M. A. (1985). "Procurement" vs. "donation"—access to tissues and organs for transplantation: Should "contracting out" legislation be adopted? *Transplantation Proceedings, 17*(6, Suppl. A), 53-68.

Winkel, F. W. (1984). Public communication on donor cards: A comparison of persuasive styles. *Social Science and Medicine, 19,* 957-963.

Youngner, S. J., Allen, M., Bartlett, E. T., Cascorbi, H. F., Hau, T., Jackson, D. L., Mahowald, M. B., & Martin, B. J. (1985). Psychosocial and ethical implications of organ retrieval. *New England Journal of Medicine, 313,* 321-324.

CHAPTER 3

SOCIAL–COGNITIVE INFLUENCES ON THE WILLINGNESS TO DONATE ORGANS

BARBARA E. NOLAN AND PATRICK J. McGRATH

Behavioral research in the organ donation field is in a nascent state. As a result, it is unknown how the beliefs and emotions of individuals interact with social influences in determining organ donation behavior. In this investigation, we studied ways social and cognitive factors would affect the willingness to donate one's own organs as well as those of a family member.

Preliminary findings have been reported in regard to social contingencies affecting organ donation behavior. Barnett, Klassen, McMinimy, and Schwarz (1987) examined the differential effects of exposing subjects to two different public service announcements. One announcement described how the decision to sign a donor card would benefit the donor (self-oriented message). The other announcement emphasized the benefits that future recipients would gain from a donor organ (other-oriented message). Whereas the other-oriented message was more readily understood, the self-oriented message was more effective in increasing willingness to donate. This finding suggested that organ donation is a goal-directed behavior and may be contingent on the type of social influences to which the individual is exposed.

In addition to social influences regarding self- versus other-gain, Belk and Austin (1987) examined how organ donation behavior was associated with self-concept. These investigators did not find a uniform pattern in the willingness to donate specific organs. Rather, willingness to donate varied according to the degree to which each organ was believed to be an integral part of the self. Subjects reported the following decremental importance of association between self-concept and organs: eyes, heart, kidneys, and liver. The investigation by Belk and Austin highlighted the importance of cognitive–affective processes in mediating the decision to donate.

Wilms, Kiefer, Shanteau, and McIntyre (1987) also suggested that the willingness to donate is contingent on emotional qualities that are attributed to specific organs. These investigators found that donors and nondonors could be separated according to ratings of sacredness, emotionality, and mysteriousness that they assigned to specific organs. Interestingly, accuracy of information about the location and function of organs did not discriminate between subjects who were willing to donate and those who were not.

We could not locate any studies that have specifically addressed how cognitive–affective processes and social situational factors might interact to influence organ donation behavior. Parisi and Katz (1986) suggested that promotional campaigns have elicited both positive and negative attitudes toward organ donation. From a survey of 110 adults, they observed that the strongest commitment toward organ donation was held by individuals who had a combination of high positive and low negative beliefs. Findings from this survey also supported the notion that negative beliefs about organ donation are prevalent among a large proportion of the general public. For example, Parisi and Katz found a high prevalence of fear that potential donors would be at risk for mutilation and inadequate provision of medical services.

These misgivings about the consequences of signing a donor card have been observed repeatedly in other investigations (Gallup Organization, 1985; Moores, Clarke, Lewis, & Mallick, 1976; Simmons, Bruce, Bienvenue, & Fulton, 1974). There is a need to determine whether providing information to offset negative beliefs will positively influence the willingness to donate organs. This study was designed to examine that issue.

The purposes of the study were (a) to determine if willingness to donate organs is enhanced by emotion-based or fact-based information or by both and (b) to ascertain if an emotion-based or a fact-based approach interacts with the willingness to donate to recipient categories that vary in the degree of personal relevance to the donor.

METHOD

Subjects
The subjects for this study were 92 English-speaking university students enrolled in a third-year developmental psychology course at an urban Canadian university. All subjects received course credit for their participation.

At the time this research was conducted, B. E. Nolan was supported by an M. R. C. doctoral studentship. P. J. McGrath was supported by a Career Scientist Award, Ontario Ministry of Health.

We wish to thank Robert Nolan for his critical review of an earlier draft of this chapter. We also want to thank our research assistant, Serena D'Costa, who volunteered many hours to code and input data for this study.

Procedure

Subjects were informed that the study was being done in conjunction with Health and Welfare Canada (the Canadian equivalent of the U.S. National Institutes of Health). The study was described as a regular 10-year update of the attitudes held by university students with regard to social and health issues. After signing an agreement to participate, each subject completed a demographic survey and a battery of six validated questionnaires. The survey included measures on the following variables: age, gender, university major, native language, drinking and smoking habits, health ratings compared with others of the same age, and presence of and perceived susceptibility to 12 major illnesses. The six questionnaires addressed a wide scope of theoretically meaningful variables. These included physical symptom reporting (Pennebaker, 1982), social desirability (Strahan & Gerbasi, 1972), religious commitment (Glock & Stark, 1973), empathy (Mehrabian & Epstein, 1972), death anxiety (Conte, Weiner, & Plutchik, 1982), and belief in a just world (Rubin & Peplau, 1975). Half of the subjects were then exposed to emotion-based information and half were exposed to fact-based information. Finally, each subject completed the Nolan Organ Donation Survey (Nolan, 1987). This survey examines attitudes and behaviors pertaining to the donation of an individual's own organs as well as those of a family member. As subjects submitted their completed forms, each one was informed that the research was not part of a Health and Welfare Canada study but was an investigation into attitudes and behaviors pertaining to organ donation.

The *emotion-based* information to which half the subjects were exposed was a personal reflection that had been published in a newsletter (Bowers, 1986–87). It was written by the mother of a 5-year-old girl who had been killed in a freak accident. The child had died several days after being hit by a piece of ice that fell from a rooftop. In the note, the mother detailed the pain she and her husband experienced during the days following the accident while their unconscious child fought for her life. The mother emotionally described the process that the parents went through in deciding to donate the child's organs. The note closed with an account of how the donation helped the parents accept their daughter's death by allowing part of her to live on in other children.

The *fact-based* condition was an information sheet issued by the federal government regarding myths typically associated with organ donation. The information sheet directly addressed issues such as the fear of mutilation, the concern that donation would interfere with the family's mourning process, and the belief that lifesaving measures would not be initiated on behalf of someone who had signed a donor card. The fact-based condition did not contain any description of personal or humanitarian benefits that could result from organ donation.

Independent judges were selected to rate the strength of the emotional and informational content in the emotion- and fact-based information sets. Ten judges were selected and randomly assigned to evaluate either the emotion- or fact-based information. The five judges in each group did not know the purpose of the study or that a second information package existed.

The degrees of emotional and informational content in the treatment conditions were assessed by using separate Likert-type scales, ranging from 1 (*not at all*) to 10 (*extremely*). An index of emotionality was calculated from the judges' ratings for each information set. This index was a difference score, which was computed by subtracting the informational content score from the emotional content score. A one-tailed t test confirmed that the emotion-based information set was more emotional than the fact-based information set, $t(9) = 2.19$, $p < .05$). The interrater reliability coefficient (r) for the emotional and informational content of the information sets was .72. Having established the efficacy of the treatment conditions, analyses proceeded.

RESULTS

Of the 92 subjects who comprised the original sample, 4 had incomplete data. The final sample ($N = 88$) was composed of 68 women and 20 men (aged 19–54 years; $M = 28.3$ years, $SD = 9.4$ years). The mean age is higher than is typical of most university samples because of 3 students in their 50s. The median age for this sample was 23.0 years.

The sample was divided into those who had previously signed organ donor cards (signers; $n = 44$) and those who had not signed cards (nonsigners; $n = 44$). Subjects were equally distributed across the emotion-based condition ($n = 44$) and fact-based condition ($n = 44$).

Analysis of Psychological Profile

A 2 (emotion- and fact-based) × 2 (signers and nonsigners) multiple analysis of variance (MANOVA) revealed no differences on the psychological variables. The following statistics were found in the MANOVA: a main effect for condition, $F(5, 78) = 0.55$; a main effect for cards, $F(5, 78) = 0.96$; and a Condition × Cards interaction, $F(5, 78) = 0.29$. Dependent measures included in this MANOVA were social desirability, religious commitment, empathy, death anxiety, and belief in a just world.

Analysis of Subjective Health Ratings

A 2 (emotion- and fact-based) × 2 (signers and nonsigners) MANOVA revealed no differences on the subjective health ratings. The Condition × Cards interaction was nonsignificant, as were the main effects for condition and cards, $F(7, 44) = 0.73$; $F(7, 44) = 1.40$; and $F(7, 44) = 0.92$, respectively. Variables included in this MANOVA were physical symptom reporting, smoking and drinking habits, and presence of and susceptibility to major diseases.

Analysis of Attitudes Toward Advertising and Legislation

A 2 (emotion- and fact-based) × 2 (signers and nonsigners) MANOVA revealed significant differences on attitudes toward advertising and legislation pertaining to organ donation. A nonsignificant interaction, $F(10, 57) = 1.35$, was found.

Significant main effects emerged for the condition variable, $F(10, 57) = 2.23$, $p < .03$, and the cards variable, $F(10, 57) = 3.00, p < .004$.

The significant multivariate F ratio for condition was accounted for by two variables at the univariate level. The first variable pertained to subjects' ratings of required request legislation (i.e., how much they favored legislation that would require physicians to ask families to donate the organs of a recently deceased loved one, regardless of the circumstances surrounding the death). The second variable was how strongly subjects agreed that physicians should approach families only if the loved one's death had been expected for a long time (death expected). Two other variables approached significance: (a) how strongly subjects felt that individuals should be allowed to specify the purposes for which their organs could be used (specify purpose) and (b) how strongly subjects felt that individuals should be allowed to advertise for an organ (advertise). The marginal means and standard deviations associated with these variables are reported in Table 1.

The means in Table 1 indicated that subjects in the fact-based condition were more opposed to required request legislation than were those in the emotion-based condition. The fact-based group was less opposed to legislation that would require physicians to approach families who had been expecting the death of a family member for a long time. It is important to note that the means for both groups indicated opposition to legislation that would require request in either of these two conditions. The means in Table 1 also indicated that fact-based subjects were less supportive of allowing donors to specify the purposes for which their organs could be used. They were also more supportive of allowing patients to advertise for organs. No differences existed between the emotion- and fact-based groups regarding their opposition toward presumed consent (i.e., the assumption that everyone is a donor unless a written statement to the contrary can be produced). The means and standard deviations for this variable were -3.00 and 2.72 and -2.56 and 2.43 for the emotion- and fact-based groups, respectively.

Table 1

MEANS AND STANDARD DEVIATIONS ASSOCIATED WITH MAIN EFFECT FOR ADVERTISING AND LEGISLATION PERTAINING TO ORGAN DONATION FOR EMOTION- AND FACT-BASED CONDITIONS

Variable	Emotion-based		Fact-based	
	M	SD	M	SD
Required request	− 1.69	3.42	− 3.84	3.15
Death expected	− 2.70	3.11	− 2.08	3.11
Specify purposes	2.91	3.38	1.51	3.53
Advertise	1.91	3.22	3.16	2.84

Note. The rating scale ranged from −5 (*strongly disagree*) to +5 (*strongly agree*) for all four ratings.

Table 2

MEANS AND STANDARD DEVIATIONS ASSOCIATED WITH MAIN EFFECT
FOR ADVERTISING AND LEGISLATION PERTAINING TO ORGAN DONATION
FOR SIGNERS AND NONSIGNERS

Variable	Signers		Nonsigners	
	M	**SD**	**M**	**SD**
Required request	− 1.34	3.49	− 3.65	2.98
Death expected	− 3.80	2.79	− 1.35	3.42
Physician chooses	2.55	2.38	1.35	2.83
How informed	2.73	0.66	1.96	0.82
Advertising if hospital unable to provide organs	0.20	3.55	1.62	2.73

Note. The rating scale ranged from −5 (*strongly disagree*) to +5 (*strongly agree*) for all four ratings.

Recall that the MANOVA examining advertising and legislation also produced a significant main effect for the cards variable. The significant multivariate F ratio for cards was accounted for by four variables at the univariate level. The means in Table 2 indicated that, compared with the signers, nonsigners were significantly more opposed to required request legislation but were less opposed to legislation in circumstances where a death had been expected. Nonsigners were significantly less supportive of allowing physicians to use their own judgment in deciding which families to approach to request an organ. In addition, nonsigners rated themselves as being less informed on organ donation issues, but more supportive of allowing individuals to advertise for organs in situations where hospitals demonstrated an inability to provide them.

It is worth noting that signers and nonsigners were both opposed to legislation that would require doctors to approach family members regardless of circumstances, as well as in cases where death has been expected for a long time. Both signers and nonsigners were opposed to presumed consent and to legislation that would require physicians to request organs from families who had suffered the sudden death of a loved one. With regard to procedures surrounding organ requests, this sample was most supportive of allowing doctors to use their own judgment in deciding which potential donor families should be approached. Finally, the means in Table 2 indicated that in regard to allowing persons to advertise for needed organs, signers were undecided on this issue and nonsigners were weakly supportive of this behavior.

Analysis of Previous Exposure to Organ Donation Issues

A 2 (emotion- and fact-based) × 2 (signers and nonsigners) MANOVA revealed differences between signers and nonsigners on their previous exposure to organ donation issues. The Condition × Cards interaction was nonsignificant, $F(4, 79)$

= 2.10. A significant main effect was found for the cards variable, $F(4, 79) = 14.88$, $p < .001$. However, no main effect emerged for condition, $F(4, 79) = 1.20$. All variables were significant at the univariate level ($p < .001$). The variables that were included in this analysis were (a) how informed subjects felt on issues pertaining to organ donation, (b) how many persons they knew who had signed organ donor cards, (c) how much they had discussed organ donation with family members, and (d) how much their family members agreed with their decision to donate.

As noted in Table 3, the means for this analysis indicated that compared with nonsigners, signers were more likely to be persons who (a) felt informed about organ donation issues, (b) knew more people who had signed a donor card, (c) discussed organ donation more frequently with their family members, and (d) had families who supported their decision to donate.

Willingness To Donate One's Own Organs

A 2 (emotion- and fact-based) × 2 (signers and nonsigners) by 3 (research, treatment, and transplant recipient categories) mixed analysis of variance (ANOVA) was conducted to determine if individuals were more likely to donate to recipient categories that were defined as more personally relevant. The recipient category was a within variable. This variable was formed by using the category breakdown that is frequently available on donor cards: research, treatment, and transplantation. These categories were of increasing personal relevance to a potential donor.

Analyses demonstrated a nonsignificant between-variables interaction, $F(1, 82) = 0.00$, and no main effect for the condition variable, $F(1, 82) = 0.10$. A main effect emerged for cards, $F(1, 82) = 7.34$, $p < .01$. The means and standard deviations associated with the marginal means for this variable were as follows: signers, $M = 3.08$, $SD = 3.16$; nonsigners, $M = 1.76$, $SD = 3.87$.

Analyses of the within variable did not reveal a Condition × Cards × Recipient interaction, $F(2, 164) = 0.35$. The two-way interaction between cards

Table 3

MEANS AND STANDARD DEVIATIONS ASSOCIATED WITH PREVIOUS
EXPOSURE TO ORGAN DONATION ISSUES FOR SIGNERS AND NONSIGNERS

Variable	Signers		Nonsigners	
	M	*SD*	*M*	*SD*
How informed	2.74	0.66	1.98	0.88
Know other consenters	1.93	1.31	0.72	1.08
Discuss with family	2.19	1.31	1.12	1.24
Family agrees with decision	8.65	2.65	6.56	1.94

Note. The rating scale ranged from −5 (*strongly oppose*) to +5 (*strongly favor*) to describe how subjects felt about the use of their organs.

and recipients was nonsignificant, $F(2, 164) = 1.01$. Similarly, the two-way interaction between the condition variable and recipient was nonsignificant, $F(2, 164) = 0.69$. A significant main effect for recipients was found, $F(2, 164) = 59.55$, $p < .001$. The marginal means and standard deviations for the recipient categories were as follows: research, $M = -1.73$ and $SD = 3.85$; treatment, $M = 3.24$ and $SD = 2.80$; and transplantation, $M = 4.28$ and $SD = 2.19$ (see Figure 1).

Post hoc comparisons using the Newman-Keuls method were conducted on the marginal means for the recipient variable. These comparisons revealed that subjects rated themselves as being significantly more willing to donate their own organs for treatment and for transplantation purposes than for research. In addition, subjects were more supportive of donating for transplantation than for treatment purposes.

Willingness To Donate Organs of a Family Member

The willingness to donate organs of a family member was investigated in a 2 (emotion- and fact-based) × 2 (signers and nonsigners) × 4 (research, stranger, acquaintance, and family recipient categories) mixed ANOVA. The recipient variable was utilized to assess subjects' willingness to donate across categories of increasing personal relevance. This variable was formed because previous research indicated that willingness to donate organs changed as a function of the personal relevance of the donor. That is, an incremental willingness to donate was found across donor categories of self, child, and another family member (cf. Gallup Organization, 1985; Prottas, 1983). The categories in this study were designed to determine if a similar phenomenon existed when the identity of the recipient was made more personally relevant. Subjects used an 11-point rating

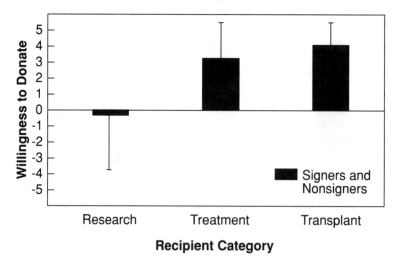

Figure 1 Effect of recipient category on willingness to donate one's own organs

scale, ranging from −5 (*strongly oppose*) to +5 (*strongly favor*), to describe how likely they would be to donate the organs of a family member to recipients in each of the four categories.

Analyses demonstrated that the Cards × Recipient interaction was significant, $F(3, 243) = 10.21, p < .001$ (see Figure 2). However, there were nonsignificant interactions for Cards × Condition × Recipient, $F(3, 243) = 0.82$, as well as for Recipient × Condition, $F(3, 243) = 0.45$. The main effect for the condition variable was also nonsignificant, $F(1, 81) = 0.29$.

The simple main effects associated with this interaction revealed that, compared with nonsigners, signers were significantly more likely to donate to recipients in the stranger and acquaintance categories. It was theoretically important that signers and nonsigners did not differ in the willingness to donate to another family member and in their unwillingness to donate to research.

Simple post hoc comparisons using Newman-Keuls indicated that signers were significantly more likely ($p < .01$) to donate to a stranger, an acquaintance, or another family member, as compared with donating to research. No significant differences emerged with regard to how likely signers were to donate to a stranger, acquaintance, or family member. Post hoc comparisons of the ratings of nonsigners revealed significant differences among all categories ($p < .01$). That is, nonsigners were significantly more likely to donate to a family member than to an acquaintance, to a stranger, or to research. They were also more likely to donate to an acquaintance than to a stranger or to research and were more likely to donate to a stranger than to research. Of interest in this analysis is the fact that even nonsigners were not opposed to donating organs to a personally relevant recipient category (also found by J. Shanteau and J. J. Skowronski; see chapter 6 in this volume).

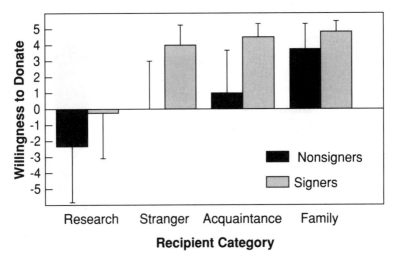

Figure 2 Effect of recipient category on willingness to donate family organs

DISCUSSION

Exposing subjects to emotion- or fact-based information exerted relatively little effect on subjects' willingness to donate their own organs or those of a family member. In particular, no differences were evident on psychological variables, subjective health ratings, or previous exposure to organ donation issues. The only differences that emerged pertained to attitudes toward legislation, with fact-based subjects being less favorably disposed toward legislation than were emotion-based subjects.

Significant differences appeared on the basis of whether subjects had previously signed an organ donor card. Compared with nonsigners, the signers felt better informed, had more family discussion about organ donation, had had more discussions about organ donation with their families, had families who agreed with their decision, knew more persons who had signed donorcards, and felt more strongly that physicians should be allowed to choose whether or not to ask families for organs. Signers and nonsigners did not differ on psychological variables, subjective health ratings, or most aspects of legislation governing the actions of physicians in requesting donor organs. Both signers and nonsigners were more willing to donate organs to recipients in categories that were more personally relevant. This pattern existed regardless of whether subjects were asked about donating their own organs or those of a family member.

The findings from this study suggest three recommendations that address distinct aspects of organ donation. The first relates to the design of future organ donor cards. The second pertains to the manner in which the procurement process is described to potential donors at the time that an organ is requested. The third recommendation addresses the need for further investigation into the use of donated organs for research purposes.

First, it is important that on all donor cards, the research category be identified as totally distinct from other categories. This is not currently done. In fact, on most donor cards, the treatment, transplantation, and research options are listed consecutively, and donors are asked to specify the conditions under which they wish their organs *not* to be used. New cards need to be designed that allow donors to sign on one line to consent to the use of their organs for treatment or transplantation and on another line to permit researchers or medical educators to have access to donated body parts.

Second, procurement programs need to highlight the procedural differences that occur when donors agree to donate for transplantation but not for research or medical education. Previous investigation (Nagy, 1985; Nolan & Spanos, 1989) has demonstrated that many persons are concerned that donating organs will interrupt the natural grieving process of the family. Although this may be true if the entire body is donated to a medical school (Nagy, 1985), it is not true when specific organs are donated.

Third, it is vital that prospective donors know that their own organs or those of a family member will be used for transplantation or treatment purposes rather than for research. It is possible that the lay public does not make this distinction, even though it appears to be an accepted fact among the medical community. An extension of this point is that further research needs to determine if donors are opposed to having *rejected* organs used for research. Organs can be deemed unsuitable for transplantation for a variety of reasons: It may be impossible to locate an appropriate recipient, or a pathological condition may be discovered in a donated organ. Several subjects in this study commented that they were opposed to their organs being used for research but would be quite willing to allow researchers to determine why a recipient had rejected their transplanted organ. Investigation needs to be conducted into the conditions under which donors might approve of research being carried out on donated organs.

References

Barnett, M. A., Klassen, M., McMinimy, V., & Schwarz, L. (1987). The role of self- and other-oriented motivation in the organ donation decision. In M. Wallendorf & P. Anderson (Eds.), *Advances in consumer research* (Vol. 14, pp. 335–337). Provo, UT: Association for Consumer Research.

Belk, R. C., & Austin, M. C. (1987). Organ donation willingness as a function of extended self and materialism. In M. van Venkatesen (Ed.), *Advances in health care research* (pp. 84–88). Toledo, OH: Association for Health Care Research.

Bowers, D. M. (1986–87). Something good happened that day. *Lifelines, 1*(4), p. 3.

Conte, H. R., Weiner, M. B., & Plutchik, R. (1982). Measuring death anxiety: Conceptual, psychometric, and factor-analytic aspects. *Journal of Personality and Social Psychology, 43*, 775–785.

Gallup Organization, Inc. (1985). *The U.S. public's attitudes toward organ transplants/ organ donation.* (G084249). Princeton, NJ: Author.

Glock, C., & Stark, R. (1973). Dimensions of religious commitment. In J. P. Robinson & P. R. Shave (Eds.), *Measures of social psychological attitudes* (rev. ed. pp. 642–649). Ann Arbor, MI: Survey Research Center, Institute for Social Research.

Mehrabian, A., & Epstein, N. (1972). A measure of emotional empathy. *Journal of Personality and Social Psychology, 40*, 525–543.

Moores, B., Clarke, C., Lewis, B. R., & Mallick, N. P. (1976). Public attitudes toward kidney transplantation. *British Medical Journal, 1*, 629–631.

Nagy, F. (1985). A model for a donated body program in a school of medicine. *Death Studies, 9*, 245–251.

Nolan, B. E. (1987). *Organ donation survey.* Unpublished manuscript, University of Ottawa, Ottawa, Canada.

Nolan, B. E., & Spanos, N. P. (1989). Psychosocial variables associated with willingness to donate organs. *Canadian Medical Association Journal, 14*, 27–32.

Parisi, N., & Katz, I. (1986). Attitudes toward posthumous organ donation and commitment to donate. *Health Psychology, 5*, 565–580.

Pennebaker, J. W. (1982). *The psychology of physical symptoms.* New York: Springer.

Prottas, J. M. (1983). Encouraging altruism: Public attitudes and the marketing of organ donation. *Health and Society, 61*, 278–306.

Rubin, A., & Peplau, L. A. (1975). Who believes in a just world? *Journal of Social Issues, 31*, 65–87.

Simmons, R. J., Bruce, J., Bienvenue, R., & Fulton, J. (1974). Who signs an organ donor card: Traditionalism versus transplantation. *Journal of Chronic Diseases*, 27, 491–502.

Strahan, R., & Gerbasi, K. C. (1972). Short, homogeneous versions of the Marlowe–Crowne Social Desirability Scale. *Journal of Clinical Psychology, 28*, 191–193.

Wilms, G., Kiefer, S. W., Shanteau, J., & McIntyre, P. (1987). Knowledge and image of body organs: Impact on willingness to donate. In M. Wallendorf & P. Anderson (Eds.), *Advances in consumer research* (Vol. 14, pp. 338–341). Provo, UT: Association for Consumer Research.

CHAPTER 4

SUBJECTIVE MEANING OF TERMS USED IN ORGAN DONATION:
ANALYSIS OF WORD ASSOCIATIONS

JAMES SHANTEAU AND KIMBERLY A. LININ

Although most adults hold favorable attitudes toward organ donation (Manninen & Evans, 1985), misconceptions persist about the donation process. Prottas (1983) observed concerns about disfigurement of the deceased, premature removal of organs, and a generalized mistrust of doctors. These misconceptions may explain, in part, why the rates of donation remain low despite widespread sympathy for the plight of potential recipients (McIntyre et al., 1987).

Many of the reported misunderstandings appear to revolve around the language of organ procurement. Common medical terms, such as *harvesting* and *brain death*, may have unintended meanings and implications for the lay population (Tiefel, 1978). If so, the choice of language by procurement professional inadvertently may contribute to unfavorable organ donation decisions.

The present research was designed to investigate subjective perceptions of various terms common in organ procurement. Subjects were asked to give open-ended word-association responses to a list of medical concepts. A particular focus here is on terms related to definitions of death—*brain death, brain-dead, heart death*, and *heart-dead*. For comparison, analyses are also included for terms for two serious but still-living conditions—*coma* and *vegetable*.

ASSOCIATIVE METHOD

Szalay and Deese (1978) described the Associative Method for collecting and analyzing word association responses. They presented a "framework and a method for the comparative study of the perceptions, attitudes, and cultural frames of reference shared by groups of people" (p. vii). They illustrated their approach by cross-cultural analyses of terms such as *hungry* and *educated.*

To avoid the problems of arbitrary interpretation of qualitative word-association responses, two procedures were used by Szalay and Deese to produce quantitative output. First, the results were analyzed at a group level so that major trends could be identified and idiosyncratic responses eliminated. Second, the responses were given weights depending on sequential order; these weighted scores were then summed to produce a numerical value for each term. These procedures allowed a quantitative analysis of a group's reactions to a term.

A major advantage of the associative approach is that it minimizes interpretations by the researcher. "It does not rely on questioning or scaling, and it is relatively free, except in the selection of stimuli, from the rationalizations and preconceptions of the investigator" (Szalay & Deese, 1978, p. ix). This is an important feature for organ donor research, where interpretations can be influenced by the wording of items or by the presence of prior information (Wilms, Kiefer, Shanteau, & McIntyre, 1987).

Szalay and Deese (1978) see an important application of their approach in understanding communication: "From a psychological point of view, communicating is largely a matter of knowing what themes are important to people and addressing those themes in ways that accord with the subjective meaning people attach to them" (p. vii). Understanding more about the language of organ procurement, therefore, may pave the way to increased rates of donation.

METHOD

Subjects

Forty-five subjects (21 women and 24 men) between the ages of 18 and 21 participated in this experiment as a partial requirement for their introductory psychology course.

Before signing up, subjects were told the study involved their current knowledge and reactions to medical terms. No mention was made of organ donation or procurement. Informed consent procedures were followed, with responses coded anonymously. Subjects were given the option of leaving the study at any time; none did. Subjects were fully debriefed.

This research was supported in part by a grant from the Bureau of General Research at Kansas State University. Preparation of the manuscript was supported by an award from the Division of Organ Transplantation, Department of Health and Human Services.

We want to thank Richard Harris and J. D. Jasper for their comments on this research. We also wish to recognize Jim Springer and Jane Warmbrodt of the Midwest Organ Bank for their support and encouragement of this project.

Correspondence concerning this chapter should be addressed to James Shanteau, Bluemont Hall, Department of Psychology, Kansas State University, Manhattan, KS 66506-5302.

Stimulus Materials

The following 14 terms and phrases were presented orally one at a time to subjects and written down on a chalkboard:

Organ donation*	Kidney transplant
Organ transplantation	Cornea (eye) transplant
Organ recipient	Vegetable (human condition)*
Organ bank	Coma*
Heart-dead*	Heart death*
Brain-dead*	Brain death*
Heart-transplant	Organ donation*

The items were selected to represent significant aspects or concepts in organ donation. Those denoted by an asterisk (*) are discussed in this report; the others were fillers.

The term *organ donation* was included both at the beginning and at the end of the list. The purpose was to see what changes might take place from participating in an organ donor study. Prior research indicated that subjects may modify their behavior during the course of an organ donation study (Wilms et al., 1987). The present results revealed that subjects produced more responses to *organ donation* at the end of the list, but that these responses were not qualitatively different from those at the beginning.

Procedure

The experiment was administered to groups of 5 to 15 subjects. After signing the informed consent form, subjects supplied demographic information about gender, age, and so forth.

The task instructions were read aloud. They stated that the experiment was "designed to measure your current knowledge and reactions to various medical and health terms." After each term was presented, subjects were to write it on a blank piece of paper; this was to ensure they understood and had a chance to think about the word(s). They were then to "begin writing—phrases, one-word responses, etc.—whatever enters your mind." They continued writing until stopped by the researcher after an elapsed time of two minutes.[1]

To encourage subjects to answer completely and honestly, they were given three guides:

1. After completing each item, they were told "not (to) go back to a term to change or add anything."
2. They were told "not (to) be inhibited in your responses—we want your initial reactions to each word."

---

1. Szalay and Deese recommend a one-minute time interval for obtaining responses. Pilot research, however, indicated that two minutes was more appropriate because of difficulties many subjects have in thinking about death-related topics.

3. It was emphasized that "there are no right or wrong answers" and that
   they should respond with "whatever enters your mind."

After completing the 14 items, subjects filled out a follow-up questionnaire
about the clarity of instructions and ease of responding to the terms. All subjects
indicated that they understood the task and could respond appropriately. They
were also asked about their willingness to sign an organ donor card. The percentages of those already signed (13%), those willing to sign if asked (29%), those
uncertain about signing (47%), those opposed to signing (9%), and others (2%)
are comparable to previous studies conducted with this subject population (Mc-
Intyre et al., 1987; see also chapter 11, by J. J. Skowronski in this volume).

Analysis

Using the associative method described by Szalay and Deese (1978), the following steps were taken in analyzing the data:[2]

1. All responses were listed in order for each subject. Any obviously
   idiosyncratic responses were eliminated, for example, "Uncle Fred."
2. Each successive response was assigned weight values as follows:

		Value			Value
First response	=	6	Sixth response	=	3
Second response	=	5	Seventh response	=	3
Third response	=	4	Eighth response	=	2
Fourth response	=	3	Ninth response	=	2
Fifth response	=	3	Tenth response	=	1

All subsequent responses were given the weight of 1. Although the scoring
system allows up to 10 or more responses, most subjects wrote down fewer
associations (see Tables 1 through 4).

The values were analyzed separately for men and women. Similar response
categories were combined, for example, "doctor" and "nurse." Any responses
listed by 10 percent or fewer subjects were eliminated. The scores for the remaining responses were computed and listed in numerical order.

Three categorical analyses were performed. First, responses were classified
by whether they were factual (e.g., "no brain activity") or emotional (e.g.,
"sad"). Second, the factual items were classified by whether they were medically
appropriate or not given the information presented; for instance, the response
"heart stops" to *heart-dead* would be considered appropriate, whereas the response "coma" would not. Third, responses were coded as implying death (e.g.,
"heart stops") or life potential (e.g., "life support"). Some responses (e.g.,
"doctor/nurse") were considered neutral and ignored in these classifications.

To check for consistency, the results for two men and two women were
reanalyzed independently several months later. Nearly identical results were ob-

---

2. A variety of other analyses were performed. The procedure suggested by Szalay and Deese,
however, produced the most meaningful and least arbitrary interpretations.

served, with over 90% reliability. The analyses were also checked by another coder unconnected with the study; again, a high degree of replicability (over 83%) was observed.[3]

RESULTS

Individual Differences

Various analyses of individual differences were performed. Several comparisons were made between subjects varying in their willingness to sign a donor card, but there were no notable trends. For instance, the percentage of responses classified as indicating potential recovery were 43%, 35%, 37%, and 37% for signed donors, willing, uncertain, and opposed subjects, respectively.

The only individual difference variable that produced any sizable effect was gender. For the most part, men and women agreed on the highest valued responses, but there were some discrepancies for associations with lower values. Accordingly, the tabled results are presented separately for men and women.

Primary Analyses

Tables 1 to 4 give the results for *brain death*, *brain-dead*, *heart death*, and *heart-dead*, respectively. All associations that met the criteria are listed. The "Score" entries are the weighted sums for each response, averaged across subjects. The "Rank" values are the order of scores for the group and for men and women separately.

Five general trends are evident from these tables. First, as indicated at the bottom of each table, subjects generated a reasonably large set of shared associations; only about one response per subject was unique. Second, even though there were gender differences, the initial responses were similar for men and women. Third, although women listed more associations, their responses were not qualitatively different from those of men. Fourth, the distribution of responses is skewed, with a few associations with high scores and many with low scores. Finally, 78.5% of the associations were factual as opposed to emotional; of these, 42.2% were medically accurate. Thus, over half of the responses were technically incorrect.

The responses in Table 1 for *brain death* present a picture of stoppage of life and mourning. Associations such as "ending of life," "no brain activity," "sad," and "funeral" provide a view of finality. The sum of scores for responses implying life was 2.82; the comparable sum for responses implying death was 5.94—a life/death ratio of .47. By (unweighted) count, 68% of the classifiable responses were indicative of being deceased. The presence of "vegetable" and

---

3. The initial coding and analyses were performed by the second author. We thank J. D. Jasper for his assistance in checking the consistency of these analyses. Because the analyses involved several steps, there was no single number that could be used to measure reliability.

Table 1

RESPONSES AND WEIGHTED SCORES TO *BRAIN DEATH* FOR MEN AND
WOMEN

All subjects		Response	Men		Women	
Rank[a]	Score[b]	category	Rank	Score	Rank	Score
1	2.13	Vegetable	1	2.16	2	2.10
2	1.78	Ending of life	2	2.04	4	1.48
3	1.69	No brain activity	3	1.04	1	2.43
4	0.96	Life support	5	0.75	7	1.19
5	0.91	Doctor/nurse	12	0.38	3	1.52
6	0.89	Death	7	0.58	6	1.23
7	0.87	Sadness	11	0.40	5	1.38
8	0.76	Hospital	10	0.46	8	1.10
9	0.71	Funeral	4	0.96	15	0.43
10	0.62	Helpless	5	0.75	13	0.48
11	0.51	Coma	8	0.50	11	0.52
12	0.44	Brain-dead	8	0.50	16	0.38
12	0.44	Accident	12	0.38	11	0.52
14	0.42	Pain and suffering	15	0.25	10	0.62
15	0.33	Hopeless	12	0.38	17	0.29
15	0.33	Legal matters			9	0.71
17	0.29	Family	16	0.13	13	0.48
	4.20	Total responses		3.29		5.24
	3.19	Responses analyzed		2.46		4.05
	1.01	Unique responses		0.83		1.19

[a]The rank order of scores for the group of subjects. [b]Sum of weighted values for each response;
entries are averaged over subjects.

"life support" high on the list, however, suggests that subjects may see some
chance of recovery.[4]

In contrast, the results for *brain-dead* are shown in Table 2. Although
medically and linguistically similar to *brain death*, there were differences in the
responses. Two out of the first three associations, "vegetable" and "life sup-

---

4. Formal statistical tests were not conducted on these qualitative results because of the
absence of an independent measure of reliability. Instead the "points of reference" described by
Szalay and Deese (1978, pp. 46–48) can be used for evaluating within-group differences. A difference
of 0.28 exceeds chance at the .05 level; a difference of .36 exceeds chance at the .01 level. All
differences discussed in this chapter surpass these values.

Table 2

RESPONSES AND WEIGHTED SCORES TO *BRAIN-DEAD* FOR MEN AND WOMEN

All subjects		Response category	Men		Women	
Rank[a]	Score[b]		Rank	Score	Rank	Score
1	2.29	Ending of life	1	2.54	3	2.00
2	2.27	Vegetable	2	2.25	1	2.30
3	1.76	Life support	3	1.71	4	1.81
4	1.56	No brain activity	5	1.12	2	2.05
5	1.60	Hopeless	3	1.71	6	1.48
6	1.20	Coma	7	0.79	5	1.67
7	0.82	Sadness	9	0.46	8	1.24
7	0.82	Legal matters	12	0.33	9	1.38
9	0.73	Death	7	0.79	11	0.67
10	0.71	Family	9	0.46	9	1.00
11	0.53	Body still works	6	0.83	15	0.19
12	0.47	Hospital	15	0.18	10	0.81
13	0.40	Doctor/nurse	13	0.29	12	0.52
14	0.53	No body function	11	0.42	14	0.29
15	0.31	Accident	14	0.21	13	0.43
	4.35	Total responses		3.54		5.29
	3.62	Responses analyzed		3.00		4.33
	0.73	Unique responses		0.54		0.96

[a]The rank order of scores for the group of subjects. [b]Sum of weighted values for each response; entries are averaged over subjects.

port," are suggestive of possible recovery. The jump of "coma" from rank 11 in Table 1 to rank 6 in Table 2 also implies survival. The sums of responses implying life and death are 5.23 and 6.27; the life/death ratio of .83 is nearly double that of brain death. In all, 43% of the (unweighted) responses indicated some chance of recovery.

A comparison of *heart death* and *heart-dead* in Tables 3 and 4 reveals a number of similarities. First on both lists is "no heartbeat," with "body is dead," "death," and "CPR/revive" near the top for each. Interestingly, "transplant" is high for both terms, although it is not clear whether this refers to the patient's being a donor or receiving a transplant. There are some gender differences for "hospital," "doctor/nurse," and "heart attack."

Table 3

RESPONSES AND WEIGHTED SCORES TO *HEART DEATH* FOR MEN AND WOMEN

All subjects		Response	Men		Women	
Rank[a]	Score[b]	category	Rank	Score	Rank	Score
1	2.71	No heartbeat	1	2.37	1	3.10
2	1.87	Heart attack	1	2.37	5	1.29
3	1.44	Transplant	3	1.58	5	1.29
4	1.18	Body is dead	5	0.87	3	1.52
5	1.07	Hospital	14	0.17	2	2.10
6	1.04	Death	3	1.58	14	0.43
7	0.84	CPR/revive	8	0.42	4	1.33
8	0.69	Doctor/nurse	12	0.25	7	1.19
9	0.64	Funeral	7	0.58	10	0.71
10	0.53	Pain	6	0.67	15	0.38
10	0.53	Family	14	0.17	8	0.95
10	0.53	Surgery	10	0.33	9	0.76
13	0.51	No blood flow	9	0.38	11	0.67
14	0.42	Emergency	13	0.21	11	0.67
15	0.38	Sadness	14	0.17	13	0.62
16	0.29	Crying	11	0.29	16	0.29
	4.35	Total responses		3.50		5.62
	3.62	Responses analyzed		3.00		4.33
	0.73	Unique responses		0.54		0.96

[a]The rank order or scores for the group of subjects. [b]Sum of weighted values for each response; entries are averaged over subjects.

Overall, the patterns in Tables 3 and 4 are comparable to *brain death* in Table 1. For instance, the sums of living and deceased associations for *heart death* are 2.28 and 7.44, with a life to death ratio of .31. The comparable sums for *heart-dead* are 2.82 and 6.53, with a life/death ratio of .43. In all, 75% of the (unweighted) responses to *heart death* and 63% of responses to *heart-dead* reflected death or mourning.

Table 4

RESPONSES AND WEIGHTED SCORES TO *HEART-DEAD* FOR MEN AND
WOMEN

All subjects		Response	Men		Women	
Rank[a]	Score[b]	category	Rank	Score	Rank	Score
1	2.64	No heartbeat	1	2.17	1	3.19
2	2.51	Body is dead	2	1.92	1	3.19
3	1.37	Death	3	1.62	5	1.10
4	1.18	CPR/revive	5	1.04	3	1.33
5	0.93	No blood flow	8	0.58	3	1.33
6	0.71	Transplant	4	1.21	16	0.14
7	0.69	Brain still alive	6	0.88	12	0.48
7	0.69	Life support	7	0.71	10	0.67
7	0.69	Family	10	0.46	7	0.95
10	0.62	Sadness	11	0.42	8	0.86
11	0.53	Hospital	17	0.13	6	1.00
12	0.49	Doctor/nurse	13	0.29	9	0.71
13	0.47	Heart attack	9	0.50	13	0.43
14	0.44	Breathing stops	16	0.17	10	0.67
15	0.38	Heart monitor/EEG	15	0.21	11	0.57
16	0.36	Pain	11	0.42	15	0.29
17	0.31	Get help	13	0.29	14	0.33
	4.51	Total responses		3.79		5.33
	3.49	Responses analyzed		2.83		4.24
	1.02	Unique responses		0.96		1.09

[a]The rank order of scores for the group of subjects. [b]Sum of weighted values for each response; entries are averaged over subjects.

Additional Analyses

The results reported so far were derived from all the subjects' responses. Because of the long tail in the response distribution, however, it is possible that the findings may have been unduly influenced by less frequent associations. To check that possibility, two additional analyses were performed.

The first analysis examined the top seven responses to each item. This eliminates any responses in the tail of the distribution. The percentages of death-consistent responses for *heart death* is 70%; *heart-dead*, 70%; *brain death*, 68%; and *brain-dead*, 55%.

The second analysis examined only the first association given by each subject to each term.[5] The percentages of death-consistent responses for *heart death* is 71%; *heart-dead*, 76%; *brain death*, 69%; and *brain-dead*, 62%.

The parallel between these various analyses is notable. Together, they suggest that *brain-dead* is perceived as more indicative of recovery than the other items. This was true no matter which portion of the response distribution was examined.

Analysis of Other Items

Although the original purpose of this chapter was to examine the four death terms, the associations for *vegetable* and *coma* are also worth investigating. As can be seen in the tables, these two words were listed frequently as responses to the death terms. It would be useful, therefore, to examine how subjects responded to these terms separately.

The same type of analysis described above was applied. The results revealed that *vegetable* was perceived as a half-dead, half-live condition with little or no hope of recovery. *Coma* was seen as similar to deep sleep with a strong potential for survival. Thus, both these terms were viewed as having connotations of the potential for life.

DISCUSSION

Three findings emerge from this study. First, the associative method produced useful and consistent results. Second, with the exception of gender, these results did not vary across demographic variables. Third, there was an unexpected difference between how subjects responded to *brain-dead* and the other items. The implications of each of these findings will be discussed in reverse order.

Perceptions of Brain-Dead

Subjects' associations to *brain-dead* suggest some chance of recovery. The results in Tables 1 and 2 reveal indications that life might continue. The high scores given to "vegetable," "life support," and "coma" are reflective of someone still alive, or at least with some potential to live.

Subjects seem to be interpreting *brain-dead* as less than terminal. One explanation is that *brain-dead* is perceived as a localized or temporary condition, with the remainder of the body still alive and capable of recovery. This is

---

5. In these analyses, idiosyncratic or unclassifiable responses, such as "family" or "hospital," were ignored. Only associations that could be categorized as relating to the concept of deceased or living were included.

plausible if *brain-dead* is viewed as meaning "dead brain." In contrast, *heart death* and *heart-dead* are perceived as death of the body.

This finding has important implications for efforts to gain a family's approval for organ donation. Because the explanation of *brain-dead* is a vital step in obtaining permission (Daly, 1982; Hessing & Elffers, 1986; Murphy, 1986), use of the term *brain-dead* may encourage an incorrect impression and a false hope of recovery.

The language of organ procurement and its impact on organ donation decisions is an area in which more research is needed. The present research provides a first step in indicating how various medical terms may be understood— or misunderstood—by the general public.

Recent studies indicate that many health professionals are uncomfortable about the process of declaring brain death (Prottas & Batten, 1988), and many hold views counter to medical or legal standards (Youngner, Landefeld, Coulton, Juknialis, & Leary, 1989). This can lead these professionals to use technical terminology as a means of coping with their uncertainty (Tiefel, 1978). Unfortunately, such terminology may contribute to miscommunication with the families of potential donors.

Individual Differences

Aside from gender differences, none of the demographic analyses produced any evidence of reliable individual differences. This is surprising for the willingness-to-be-a-donor variable; other studies have reported sizable differences between those willing to be donors and those opposed (e.g., McIntyre et al., 1987; see also chapter 6 by J. Shanteau & J. J. Skowronski in this volume and chapter 11 by J. J. Skowronski in this volume). It would appear that perception of medical terms is not related to willingness to donate.

On the other hand, there were differences observed between men and women. For instance, women gave more associations to the organ donation terms. The associations given by men, however, were not qualitatively different from women; instead, women's responses subsumed those given by men. This may arise because women are more verbally articulate or because men are more reticent about describing their feelings.

Another difference between men and women can be seen in the scores for some responses. Across all items, women were more likely to mention "doctor/nurse," "sadness," and "hospital." Men, on the other hand, were more likely to respond "death," "helpless," and "hopeless."

In almost all cases, these differences are greatest for items in the lower portion of the tables. Men and women generally agreed on the responses at the top of the tables. That means there is consensus on the primary associations, with disagreement on secondary associations.

This pattern of agreement on more frequent responses and disagreement on less frequent responses may explain the mixed reports of gender effects in previous research. Some studies have observed notable gender differences; Royster, Tetreault, and Shanteau (1987) described gender effects for death anxiety, and Wilms et al. (1987) found differences between men's and women's images of body organs. Other studies, however, have not found any gender differences in how organ donation decisions are made (McIntyre et al., 1987). It may be that gender differences are most likely to show up in analyses of secondary variables.

Associative Method

These results demonstrate the usefulness of the associative method of Szalay and Deese (1978). As shown here, this approach produced reliable and interpretable results for responses to organ procurement terms.

It is significant that a few associations consistently led to high scores. Initially, we were unsure whether this approach was capable of yielding new insights into organ donation decisions. Indeed, we are unaware of any previous analyses of word associations in organ donation.

It should be noted that scoring of word associations is time-consuming. However, the associative method provided considerable return for the effort. Aside from the scoring procedure developed by Szalay and Deese (1978), we explored several other analytic methods. For the work involved, these alternative analyses produced few insights. Based on this experience, our recommendation for researchers is to carefully consider using the associative method.

References

Daly, K. (1982). The diagnosis of brain death: Overview of neurosurgical nursing responsibilities. *Journal of Neurosurgical Nursing, 4*, 85–89.

Hessing, D. J., & Elffers, H. (1986). Attitude toward death, fear of being declared dead too soon, and donation of organs after death. *Omega, 17*, 115–126.

Manninen, D., & Evans, R. (1985). Public attitudes and behavior regarding organ donation. *Journal of the American Medical Association, 253*, 3111–3115.

McIntyre, P., Barnett, M. A., Harris, R. J., Shanteau, J., Skowronski, J., & Klassen, M. (1987). Psychological factors influencing decisions to donate organs. In M. Wallendorf & P. Anderson (Eds.), *Advances in consumer research* (Vol. 14). Provo, UT: Association of Consumer Research.

Murphy, P. (1986, July). When a non-death occurs. *Nursing*, pp. 34–39.

Prottas, J. (1983). Encouraging altruism: Public attitudes and the marketing of organ donation. *Health and Society, 61*, 278–306.

Prottas, J., & Batten, H. L. (1988). Health professionals and hospital administrators in organ procurement: Attitudes, reservations, and their resolutions. *American Journal of Public Health, 78*, 642–645.

Royster, B., Tetreault, P., & Shanteau, J. (1987). *Death anxiety, social desirability, and gender differences: Influences on organ donation*. Paper presented at the meeting of the Midwestern Psychological Association, Chicago, IL.

Szalay, L. B., & Deese, J. (1978). *Subjective meaning and culture: An assessment through word associations*. Hillsdale, NJ: Erlbaum.

Tiefel, H. O. (1978, December). The language of medicine and morality. *Hastings Center Report*, pp. 11–13.

Wilms, G., Kiefer, S., Shanteau, J., & McIntyre, P. (1987). Knowledge and image of body organs: Impact on willingness to donate. In M. Wallendorf & P. Anderson (Eds.), *Advances in consumer research* (Vol. 14). Provo, UT: Association of Consumer Research.

Youngner, S. J., Landefeld, S., Coulton, C. J., Juknialis, B. W., & Leary, M. (1989). "Brain death" and organ retrieval: A cross-sectional survey of knowledge and concepts among health professionals. *Journal of the American Medical Association, 261,* 2205–2210.

CHAPTER 5

DEATH ATTITUDES AND HUMOR:
TAKING A DIFFERENT PERSPECTIVE ON ORGAN DONATION

ROBERT SHEPHERD AND HERBERT M. LEFCOURT

In contrast to the pragmatic goals of many researchers entering the field of organ donation, research at the University of Waterloo, Ontario, Canada, concerning organ donation has come about somewhat indirectly. Initially our aim was to investigate coping responses to stress within the domain of death attitudes and to explore the relation between cognitions, affect, and behaviors that arise in death-salient contexts. For example, based on results of an initial pilot study (Shepherd, 1988), we have hypothesized that higher levels of mood disturbance experienced in death-related situations are associated with a negative evaluation of death and with the avoidance of such death-salient contexts.

Although we surmised that the stress of thinking about death does have an impact on subjects' feelings and behaviors, we realized that there exists a range of reactions that can be anticipated among different persons. It has long been known that the measurable effects of stress on feelings and behaviors are often less than impressive (Johnson & Sarason, 1979; Rabkin & Struening, 1976). Research on stress and coping has suggested a variety of subject characteristics that may influence the relation between stress and distress (i.e., Cohen & Syme, 1985; Kobasa, 1979; Lefcourt, Miller, Ware, & Sherk, 1981). Of particular relevance to our own research have been results from a series of studies by Lefcourt and Martin (1986), which provided evidence that humor is a valid coping response that appears to reduce the negative impact of stressful experiences. Later studies by Porterfield (1987) and Nezu, Nezu, and Blissett (1988) have also offered support to the belief that humor somehow mitigates negative affect.

Psychologists have long speculated on the benefits of humor. For example, Freud described humor as the highest of the defense mechanisms (Freud, 1960). Frankl (1963) has argued that humor is an essential aspect of self-detachment, and therapists have since offered countless anecdotal accounts attesting to humor's ability to provide insight and a sense of proportion and to reduce tension (Block, Browning, & McGrath, 1983; Grotjahn, 1971). Thus, laughter may permit us to take perspective on the more solemn aspects of existence, such as death, and reduce the discomfort aroused by the contemplation of death-related issues, such as signing an organ donation form. To test this hypothesis, we focused our attention in a subsequent study upon the relation between humor and death attitudes (Shepherd, 1988).

In this study, we used a variety of methods to assess subjects' sense of humor. For example, Martin and Lefcourt's (1983) Situational Humor Response Questionnaire (SHRQ) assesses how often and to what degree individuals find amusement in a range of situations in which they would be at least mildly surprised or aroused, if not embarrassed or angered. In addition to using the SHRQ, we devised exercises that might provide additional data regarding subjects' sense of humor. For example, we had subjects sort a variety of cartoons selected from *New Yorker* magazine, Gary Larson's *The Far Side*, James Unger's *Herman*, and Tom Wilson's *Ziggy*. We predicted that the preference for more absurd or ironic comic styles characteristic of *New Yorker* cartoons or those in Larson's *The Far Side* would be negatively related to avoidant behaviors.

For another approach to the assessment of humor, we videotaped subjects as they made up 3-minute comedy routines. Judges later rated subjects' improvisations for the total number of witty remarks as well as overall wittiness of the story. We expected that lower ratings on this task would also be associated with more avoidant behaviors.

For our dependent measure, we felt that subjects' decision to sign an organ donor form provided an excellent example of their willingness to confront or avoid death. The appeal of the donor form as a measure of this willingness also lay in its relevance to our typical sample population—college students for whom the decision to donate was pertinent, meaningful, and actively encouraged through the inclusion of donor forms on provincial driver's licenses. To obtain information about organ donation, we interviewed subjects briefly regarding signing behavior and their willingness to donate various organs (based on a list provided by Manninen & Evans, 1985).

This research was supported in part by SSHRC Awards 453-87-0468 to the first author and 410-87-0255 to the second author. Correspondence concerning this chapter should be addressed to Robert Shepherd, Department of Psychology, University of Waterloo, Waterloo, Ontario, Canada, N2L 3G1.

Table 1

PEARSON CORRELATIONS: HUMOR SCORES AND DONOR FORM DATA.
STUDY 1

	Willing to sign donor form	Willing to donate organs
SHRQ	.20	.10
Witty comments in comedy routine	.42**	.30
Overall wittiness of comedy routine	.44**	.38*

Note. SHRQ = Situational Humor Response Questionnaire. Donor form appears on provincial driver's license.
*$p < .05$. **$p < .01$.

The results of this study are briefly summarized in Tables 1 and 2. As can be seen in Table 1, scores on the SHRQ are weakly correlated with the willingness to sign an organ donation form and with willingness to donate a number of organs; also, correlations between donor form behavior and ratings on the improvisations reveal a number of significant findings. Generally speaking, witty comments and overall wittiness scores were positively related to the willingness to sign an organ donation form and, to a somewhat lesser extent, to donate a variety of organs.

Additional evidence linking humor to favorable attitudes toward organ donation is provided by our measures based on the cartoon ratings. As seen in Table 2, preferences for the various cartoon categories were in many cases significantly related to donor form behavior. For example, in the case of willingness to sign an organ donor form, preference ratings for both *The Far Side* and *New Yorker* cartoons showed positive correlations; the correlation between ratings of *New Yorker* cartoons and donor form signing was significant at the .05 level ($r = .36$). It is interesting to note that for their humor, these cartoons rely on an appreciation for more biting social commentary and the dismantling of our human-centered superiority complex over the universe—an orientation we have since labeled *perspective-taking humor*. On the other hand, *Herman* and *Ziggy* cartoons rely on portrayals of aggressive one-upmanship in society and sympathy with a "loser." Higher ratings for either of the latter cartoons were negatively correlated with donor form signing, with the correlation between ratings of *Ziggy* and donor form signing significant at the .05 level ($r = .37$). Similar results are evident in the relation between the various cartoon ratings and subjects' willingness to donate more than one organ.[1]

1. It has been suggested that the latter relations may be a function of higher socioeconomic status, a variable common to both favorable attitudes toward donation and to admiration of cartoons such as those in the *New Yorker*. However, our results concerning actual humor production suggest that this is not sufficient to account for the relations observed.

Table 2

PEARSON CORRELATIONS: CARD SORT RATINGS AND DONOR FORM DATA. STUDY 1

Rating	Donor Form	#Organs
The Far Side	.24	.27
Ziggy	− .37*	− .29
Herman	− .19	− .34*
New Yorker	.36*	.38*

*$p < .05$.

THE NEED FOR A MORE COMPREHENSIVE APPROACH

In subsequent research, we have used the results of these first studies to construct a theoretical network of relations between death-salient cognitions, affect, behavior, and sense of humor. While the studies described here do discuss relations between all these variables, a comprehensive theory has been lacking that would relate the various components of death attitudes (in addition to avoidant or confronting behaviors) to humor. The result of our attempt to integrate death attitudes and humor is represented in Figure 1. Briefly, we see cognitions to be related primarily to the affective response to death, which, in turn, serves as an intervening variable that is directly related to behaviors. Affect is also hypothesized to mediate the relation between humor and behavior.

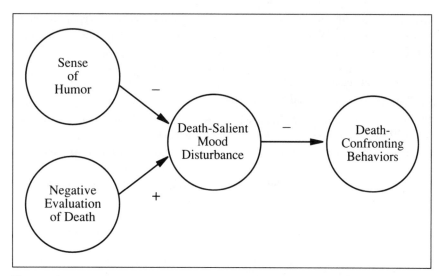

Figure 1 Hypothesized relations between sense of humor, negative evaluation of death, death-salient mood disturbance, and death-confronting behaviors.

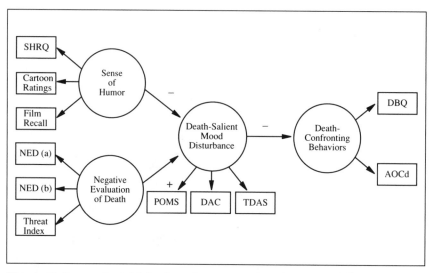

Figure 2 Structural model for first of a recent series of studies. SHRQ = Situational Humor Response Questionnaire. NED = negative evaluation of death scale. POMS = Profile of Mood States. DAC = death affect checklist. TDAS = Templer's Death Anxiety Scale. DBQ = Death Behavior Questionnaire. AOCd = Avoidance of the Ontological Confrontation of Death (Thauberger, 1979).

In order to assess this general model, we have found it necessary to use a variety of methods in what has turned out to be a three-stage process. For example, as a first step, we carried out a study on 61 undergraduate psychology students. Figure 2 provides a schematic of this study, indicating the measures used and the network of interrelations to be tested.

Several of the measures identified in Figure 2 have been briefly discussed previously. In the case of our assessment of behavior, note that rather than focus on organ donation per se, we introduced a Death Behavior Questionnaire (DBQ), which consists of questions about a number of death-related behaviors, including donor form attitudes. For each of the remaining constructs, we included several preliminary measures in addition to the established measures used in previous studies. The former included a negative evaluation of death scale (NED), designed to complement the Threat Index (Neimeyer, Dingemans, & Epting, 1977). To evaluate mood states, a death affect checklist (DAC)[2] was included along with Templer's Death Anxiety Scale (TDAS; Templer, 1970) and the Profile of Mood States (POMS; Lorr & McNair, 1982). The latter was used to assess affect subsequent to completion of these death-related questionnaires.

In addition to some of the humor measures already discussed (SHRQ and cartoon ratings), we included a new humor exercise in which subjects viewed a

---

2. The DAC was intended to assess one's affective reaction to death as a trait-like quality, as opposed to the more state-oriented POMS.

short excerpt from a humorous film, the plot of which focuses primarily on the visit of "the Grim Reaper" to a dinner party. After viewing the film, subjects were requested to recall as many humorous parts of the film as they could on paper.

Results of this study proved useful in a variety of ways. Most importantly, we were able to assess the reliability and validity of the many scales used in the study and the overall soundness of our model. These results were crucial to the design of subsequent studies.

For example, having some understanding of our measures and their adequacy, we next set out to construct a measure that specifically tapped perspective-taking humor, as it was apparent that this was a serious shortcoming in our humor battery. Using a sample of 30 undergraduates, we were able to generate a reliable and valid measure of this construct.

Furthermore, by gathering together revised measures from our first study, we used a parallel design on a larger sample ($n = 88$). In this final study, several changes were made in addition to the fine-tuning of scales. For example, to discern whether self-reported mood differed from general mood states, we obtained both pre- and postmanipulation mood assessments from subjects. We also devised a "death exercise" that allowed us to actually observe and record the incidence of death-confronting behaviors. Drawing from the work of several researchers (Handal, 1969; Sabatini & Kastenbaum, 1973; Thauberger, 1979), we constructed a series of tasks whose completion required confrontation with relevant and death-salient issues. We hoped the latter exercises would elicit strong affective reactions in most subjects.

Since our hypotheses place increasing emphasis on donor form signing as a death-confronting behavior, we believed it was important to focus on the topic of organ donation by providing subjects with an opportunity to fill out an organ donor form. To increase the salience of such a decision and cause subjects to reflect seriously upon this request, we provided an essay composed of several factual arguments in favor of organ donation. In creating such an essay, we strove to ensure that the arguments focused on potential benefits to the individual making the donation, as well as benefits accrued by recipients (see Skowronski, 1987). More generally, we emphasized prodonation attitudes and discredited antidonation beliefs (see Parisi & Katz, 1986).

We believe that this study is a logical extension of the methods used in our lab over the past several years. Although a thorough discussion of the analyses and results is beyond the scope of this chapter, we hope we have succeeded in outlining our somewhat unique theoretical approach to the issue of organ donation.

CONCLUDING REMARKS

While this chapter has represented a condensed summary of several studies on death attitudes and humor, our main intent has been to describe a theoretical approach whose purpose goes beyond the procurement of organs for transplantation purposes. The relevant features of this program include the following:

1. In selecting a dependent variable, we have found it helpful to focus not only upon organ donation, but also to consider the general case of death-confronting behaviors, around which we have built a theoretical network of relations. Although many would agree that organ procurement is a worthy social cause, we are convinced that the division of individuals into categories such as pro- or antidonation unnecessarily restricts the scope and potential benefits of psychological research in this field. In our own work, donation-related acts are strongly associated with numerous other death-related behaviors. Thus, the question of ultimate interest may not be why individuals do or do not sign organ donation forms but rather what factors explain the propensity of some individuals to confront death, whereas others appear to actively avoid the topic. The latter is of import not only to prospective donors, but also to family members whose consent is required and to those health professionals who must raise the issue of organ donation on a daily basis.

2. Researchers would be well advised not to focus exclusively on cognitive variables when conducting work in this field. One need not be a psychologist to realize that the topic of organ donation is an extremely emotional issue, particularly for bereaved family members asked to give their consent following the death of the potential donor. It is thus not surprising that many individuals appear to have required little thought in coming to a decision, whether it be in favor of or opposition to donation.

3. Individual difference variables are of import. If humor is related to organ donation, then we cannot help but speculate about other potentially relevant variables. To give some examples, death attitude research is prone to gender differences (Schulz, 1978; Templer & Ruff, 1971), which appear to have affected many of our own results. Others have speculated on the role played by altruism; the hesitancy of procurement agencies to offer financial or other incentives for organs appears to reflect an appreciation for the importance of this variable. It is only when we begin to look beyond the abstract and often irrelevant ideas people hold regarding organ donation and consider those traits which affirm us as individuals that we can fully elaborate the motivations involved in this most personal issue.

4. Finally, we must consider the role played by values in our research. Can we distinguish between efforts intended to clarify the factors involved in the decision to donate one's organs and efforts to convince more people to donate organs? And even if we desire merely a confirmation of theory, can we continue to ignore the fact that all this theorizing is heavily value-laden and may reflect our own peculiar attitudes toward death and dying? It would seem that the issue of organ donation brings us face to face with the paradox. On one hand, the ability

to consider our personal death, or that of a significant other, without severe emotional stress would seem a prerequisite of voluntary confrontation with death-related issues. Yet it is the horror that death arouses in us that drives our medical machine in its search for organ donations to forestall mortality.

References

Block, S., Browning, S., & McGrath, G. (1983). Humor in group psychotherapy. *British Journal of Medical Psychology, 56*, 89–97.

Cohen, S., & Syme, S. L. (1985). Issues in the study and application of social support. In S. Cohen and S. L. Syme (Eds.), *Social support and health* (pp. 3–22). Toronto: Academic Press.

Frankl, V. E. (1963). *Man's search for meaning.* New York: Washington Square Press.

Freud, S. (1960). *Jokes and their relation to the unconscious.* New York: Norton.

Grotjahn, M. (1971). Laughter in group psychotherapy. *International Journal of Group Psychotherapy, 21,* 234–238.

Handal, P. (1969). The relationship between subjective life expectancy, death anxiety and general anxiety. *Journal of Clinical Psychology, 25,* 38–42.

Hayduk, L. A. (1987). *Structural equation modeling with LISREL.* Baltimore: Johns Hopkins University Press.

Johnson, J. H., & Sarason, I. G. (1979). Moderator variables in life stress research. In I. G. Sarason & C. D. Spielberger (Eds.), *Stress and anxiety* (Vol. 6). Washington, DC: Hemisphere.

Jorskog, K. G., & Sorbom, D. (1984). *LISREL VI: User's guide.* Chicago: National Educational Resources.

Kobasa, S. C. (1979). Stressful life events, personality, and health: An inquiry into hardiness. *Journal of Personality and Social Psychology, 37,* 1–11.

Lefcourt, H. M., & Martin, R. A. (1986). *Humor and life stress.* New York: Springer-Verlag.

Lefcourt, H. M., Miller, R. S., Ware, E. E., & Sherk, D. (1981). Locus of control as a modifier of the relationship between stressors and moods. *Journal of Personality and Social Psychology, 41,* 357–369.

Lorr, M., & McNair, D. M. (1982). *Manual for the Profile of Mood States—bipolar form.* San Diego: Educational & Testing Service.

Manninen, D. L., & Evans, R. W. (1985). Public attitudes and behavior regarding organ donation. *The Journal of the American Medical Association, 253*(21), 3111–3115.

Martin, R. A., & Lefcourt, H. M. (1983). Sense of humor as a moderator of relation between stressors and moods. *Journal of Personality and Social Psychology, 45*(6), 1313–1324.

Neimeyer, R. A., Dingemans, P. M. A. J., & Epting, F. R. (1977). Convergent validity, situational stability and meaningfulness of the threat index. *Omega, 8*(3), 251–265.

Nezu, A. M., Nezu, C. M., & Blissett, S. E. (1988). Sense of humor as a moderator of the relation between stressful events and psychological distress: A prospective analysis. *Journal of Personality and Social Psychology, 54,* 520–525.

Parisi, N., & Katz, I. (1986). Attitudes toward posthumous organ donation and commitment to donate. *Health Psychology, 5*(6), 565–580.

Porterfield, A. L. (1987). Does sense of humor moderate the impact of life stress on psychological and physical well-being? *Journal of Research in Personality, 21,* 306–317.

Rabkin, J. G., & Struening, E. L. (1976). Life events, stress, and illness. *Science, 194,* 1013–1020.

Sabatini, P., & Kastenbaum, R. (1973). The do-it-yourself death certificate as a research technique. *Life-Threatening Behavior, 3*, 20–32.

Schulz, R. (1978). *The psychology of death, dying and bereavement.* Menlo Park: Addison-Wesley.

Shepherd, R. (1988). *Death attitudes and humor: Preliminary investigations.* Unpublished masters thesis, University of Waterloo, Waterloo, Ontario, Canada.

Skowronski, J. J. (1987). *Psychological factors influencing decisions to donate organs.* Paper presented at the meeting of the Midwestern Psychological Association.

Templer, D. I. (1970). The construction and validation of a death anxiety scale. *The Journal of General Psychology, 82*, 165–177.

Templer, D., & Ruff, C. (1971). Death anxiety scale means, standard deviations and embedding. *Psychological Reports, 29*, 173–174.

Thauberger, P. C. (1979). The avoidance of the ontological confrontation of death: A psychometric research scale. *Essence, 3*(1), 9–12.

CHAPTER 6

THE DECISION TO DONATE ORGANS:
AN INFORMATION–INTEGRATION ANALYSIS

JAMES SHANTEAU AND JOHN J. SKOWRONSKI

The purpose of the research reported in this chapter is to use a decision-making approach to evaluate subjects' willingness to donate organs. Specifically, Information Integration Theory (IIT) was applied to determine how various pieces of information combined to influence donation judgments. This approach (see Anderson, 1981, 1982) provides for simultaneous determination of combination rules and parameter estimates. Thus, it is possible both to evaluate how various pieces of information combine to influence organ donation and to assess the psychological values of that information.

In this research, the willingness to donate organs was investigated as a function of four variables: (a) whether the donor was alive or deceased at the time of donation, (b) the relatedness of the transplant recipient (relative, friend, or stranger), (c) what organ or tissue was to be donated, and (d) the prior commitment of the subject to be an organ donor (ranging from signing a card to opposition). These variables were studied using factorial designs to create systematically different stimulus—subject conditions.

Two experiments were conducted. The first, at Kansas State University, was a preliminary analysis of the effect of three stimulus factors: living–deceased donor, relatedness of recipient, and organ or tissue to be donated. The second experiment, at Ohio State University, allowed a detailed analysis of these three factors for four groups of subjects who varied on their prior willingness to be a signed organ donor.

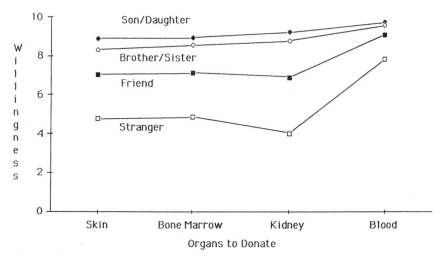

Figure 1 Mean willingness to donate various organs to relatives and strangers, while living (Experiment 1).

EXPERIMENT 1

Method

A sample of 137 undergraduates at Kansas State University completed a questionnaire containing, among other things, an IIT analysis of organ donation decisions. There were 68 men and 69 women; however, no consistent gender differences in the results were observed. Only the findings pertaining to the IIT analyses will be described here (for a description of the remaining results, see McIntyre, Barnett, Harris, Shanteau, Skowronski, & Klassen, 1987).

Although students are not necessarily representative of the larger population, they are appropriate as a target population for donation research for three reasons: (a) they are at an age when their own organs are ideal for transplantation, (b) they are more likely to engage in activities that place them at risk of fatal accidents, and (c) they have the potential for making organ donation decisions for three generations—themselves, their children, and their parents.

Two factorial designs were used: a 4 × 4 (Organ to Donate × Relatedness) design for donation while living, and a 11 × 2 (Organ to Donate × Relatedness)

This research was supported in part by a grant from the Bureau of Graduate Research at Kansas State University. Preparation of the manuscript was supported by an award from the Division of Organ Transplantation of the Public Health Service, U.S. Department of Health and Human Services.

We want to thank Pat McIntyre for her help in the initial phases of this research.

Correspondence concerning this chapter should be addressed to James Shanteau, Department of Psychology, Bluemont Hall, Kansas State University, Manhattan, Kansas 66506.

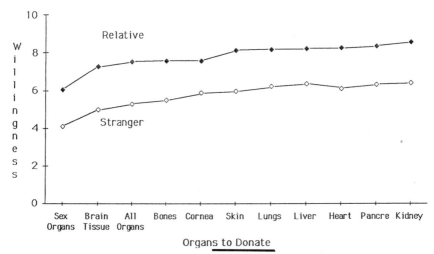

Figure 2 Mean willingness to donate various organs to relatives and strangers, after death (Experiment 1).

design for donation after death. The levels used in each design are listed in Figures 1–5. The order of presentation within each factorial was random, with the living condition presented first.

The subjects were given the following instructions: "This section concerns your willingness to donate different types of organs to different people when you are living or dead. For each of the situations described below, please indicate your willingness by using the following scale:" In the 10-point scale, 1 = *highly unwilling to donate*, 5 = *neutral*, and 10 = *highly willing to donate*. For each stimulus combination, subjects wrote down their willingness to donate next to the stimulus description.

The experiment was administered to groups of 20 to 25 subjects. Every subject made a single judgment of each stimulus combination. In contrast to most IIT studies, there were no practice trials, filler stimuli, instruction checks, or other methodological precautions.

Due to these limitations, the results reported herein are based entirely on group data. Also, as this was a preliminary study, only descriptive statistics are reported.

Results

As shown in the graphs in Figures 1, 2, and 3, the patterns of results are quite orderly. In Figure 1, the mean willingness-to-donate results for the 4 × 4 donation-while-living design are plotted. There are three notable findings. First, except for blood donation, there is relatively little difference in donation willingness across organ or tissue type; the flatness of the lines indicates that subjects were about equally likely to donate skin, bone marrow, or a kidney. Second, the relatedness of the donor is clearly important, with greater willingness to donate to a child or a sibling and less willingness to donate to a friend or a stranger. Third, the results for blood donation indicate a high degree of willingness to donate under all situations.

The results for donation likelihood after death, shown in Figure 2, reveal several noteworthy patterns. Regardless of the organ, subjects were about 20 percent more willing to donate to a relative than to a stranger. With the exception of sex organs and brain tissue, subjects were less willing to donate "all organs" than they were to donate each organ or tissue separately. Finally, there were slight but consistent differences across organs in willingness to donate—kidneys received the highest ratings and sex organs the lowest.

To contrast living and deceased conditions, Figure 3 presents the willingness to donate for comparable situations. Only those organs that can be donated both while living and deceased were considered. Also, the son or daughter and brother or sister results were combined into a single "relative" category for living donation. Several unexpected results emerged. The willingness to donate to a relative is greater while living than deceased. The opposite is true, however, for donating to strangers. Moreover, the difference between relative and stranger is roughly twice as large for living donations.

EXPERIMENT 2

The purposes of the second study were, first, to conduct a replication of Experiment 1 using a larger and somewhat older sample of subjects; second, to examine the effect of prior commitment to be an organ donor on the results; and third, to conduct statistical analysis to verify the descriptive findings from Experiment 1.

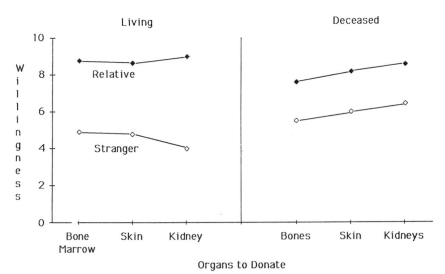

Figure 3 Mean willingness to donate various organs to relatives and strangers, while living and after death (Experiment 1).

Method

A sample of 243 night-school students at Ohio State University completed the same research materials described in Experiment 1. Four groups of subjects were defined by their willingness to sign an organ donor card. "Donors" had already signed their licenses ($n = 53$). "Favorable" subjects were willing to sign if asked ($n = 51$). "Uncertain" subjects had yet to make up their minds ($n = 113$). "Antidonation" subjects had decided not to sign ($n = 26$).

The procedure was identical to that for the first study, except that a different experimenter was used.

Results

The overall data for living donation is shown in Figure 4. These results are remarkably similar to Figure 1 from Experiment 1. Side-by-side comparisons of the overall results for deceased donation also revealed small differences between the two experiments.

Several analyses were conducted of the effects across the four donor groups. As shown in Figure 5 for the living-donation design, there were both notable similarities and differences between the groups.

First, there are clear between-group differences, $F(3, 240) = 6.72$, all $ps < .05$—with a systematic decline in willingness ratings from donors to antidonation subjects. The difference is reflected in an expanding separation of curves for the transplant recipient, with the difference between relatives and strangers increasing from donors to antidonation subjects; this was reflected by a significant Relation $\times$ Group interaction, $F(9, 720) = 7.46$.

Second, the same general ordering of results was observed across all groups; for example, the two-way Organ $\times$ Donor Group interaction and the three-way

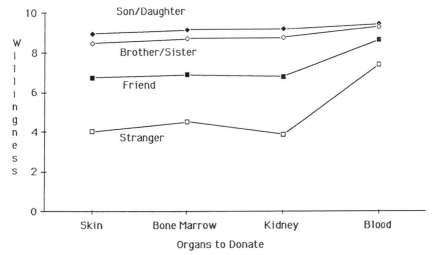

Figure 4 Mean willingness to donate various organs to relatives and strangers, while living (Experiment 2).

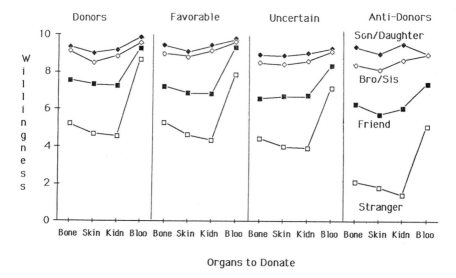

Figure 5 Mean willingness to donate various organs to relatives and strangers as a function of four groups, while living (Experiment 2).

interaction were both nonsignificant. There was a small but consistent difference between organs and tissues, with blood clearly receiving higher willingness ratings, $F(3, 720) = 92.33$.

Third, there was almost no difference across groups in their willingness to donate to relatives. Indeed, the antidonation group was as willing to donate organs to their children as the signed donor group. What distinguishes the four groups is not their willingness to donate to relatives, but rather their willingness to donate to nonrelatives.

Analyses were conducted for willingness to donate after death for the four groups. Because of the large number of data points, a plot of all four groups could not be included. However, several relevant results were apparent from the graphical and statistical analyses.

There were notable differences between groups that showed up in several ways:

1. There was a significant group difference, with steadily declining willingness to donate across groups, $F(3, 239) = 65.91$.
2. The differences between willingness to donate to relatives and strangers increased markedly across groups, $F(3, 239) = 28.69$. Signed donors, for instance, were almost as willing to donate to strangers as to relatives. However, antidonation subjects were unwilling to donate to strangers under any circumstance.
3. The relation between organ type and relatedness of recipient changed across groups. This was reflected in a significant three-way interaction, $F(30, 2390) = 2.19$.

GENERAL DISCUSSION

Consistent results were obtained from these two experiments. There does appear to be a "cognitive algebra" underlying organ donation decisions. Despite less than optimal experimental conditions, the IIT approach proved useful in revealing previously unreported patterns of behavior. These results have several implications for organ donation behavior.

Living Donation

Probably the most notable result from Experiment 1 (replicated in Experiment 2) were the patterns for living–deceased and relative–stranger. Subjects were more willing to donate to relatives while living and to strangers after death. Although the results for strangers is not surprising, the results for relatives were unexpected. Why should someone be more willing to donate to a relative while alive than after death?

One possible explanation is that the earthly rewards for being a donor can only be experienced while living, not after death. With a relative, a donation would directly benefit a known other person. If a close relative's life is saved, then the donor would still be alive to share in the experience. A donation after death cannot produce a similar experience. Therefore, the opportunity to see the rewards of donation may provide an added motivation.

Another explanation is that a request for a living donation to a relative may lead to a nearly automatic positive decision. As noted by Wilms, Kiefer, Shanteau, and McIntyre (1987), people under such circumstances think little about their behavior—living donors respond that "it was simply the right thing to do" and "I gave it no thought, I just did it." Similarly, those who donate a kidney while living reported "there was nothing to think about" and "it was the natural thing to do" (Fellner & Marshall, 1981). This suggests that such donations may be viewed rather differently than donations after death.

All Versus Separate Organs

Another finding from Experiment 1, also replicated in Experiment 2, deserves comment. There is a slight tendency to be less willing to donate all organs than to donate each of the organs separately. This implies that a request for specific organs may be treated more favorably than a request for all organs. Perhaps, subjects are unsure about what "all organs" includes and hence are less willing to donate. Whatever the reason, a request for specific organs could lead to higher rates of agreement.

Group Differences

The most notable result from Experiment 2 concerns the differences and similarities among the four groups. Unexpectedly, all groups were equally willing to donate organs to relatives while living. Even the antidonation subjects gave high willingness ratings for donation—the results for relatives are virtually indistinguishable across the four groups.

Where the groups differed was in their willingness to donate to strangers. Signed donors, on the one hand, were quite willing to donate to friends and gave intermediate ratings for strangers. Antidonation subjects, on the other hand, were very unwilling to donate to strangers and gave intermediate ratings for friends. Even blood donation for antidonation subjects was rated low for strangers.

Antidonation Subjects?

The preceding results show that under appropriate circumstances, nearly everyone was willing to be an organ donor. As long as the recipient was a child or a sibling, all groups were highly willing to donate. What separates the four groups is their willingness to donate to strangers. Committed donors are more willing to donate to strangers than are the antidonation subjects.

This means that the antidonation group is probably misnamed. They are not uniformly antidonation. Rather, they are antistranger. Under appropriate circumstances—where a close relative is the recipient—they are in fact willing to donate.

Thus, such subjects will part with organs when the perceived beneficiary is direct and identifiable. It would appear, therefore, that "antidonation" subjects are not necessarily less empathic, caring, or altruistic than others.

Increasing Donor Rates

An important implication from these results is that an effort to increase rates of donation by education is unlikely to succeed. Almost everyone is already willing to be a donor—under the right circumstances. Other studies have consistently shown that nearly all respondents are familiar with the need for more organs and are sympathetic with the plight of would-be recipients (Manninen & Evans, 1985).

Instead, the key may lie in broadening the class of those considered to be relatives or "family." One goal might be to reduce the perceived distance between insiders and outsiders. Appeals might state, for instance, that the lives saved through organ donation could be those of your neighbors; the person's life you save may be someone like yourself. This is clearly an issue that deserves additional research.

Conclusions

In summary, there are five conclusions worth noting. First, the organ shortage remains crucial, especially in light of the increasing effectiveness of transplantation technology. Efforts at resolving this need by educating the public about the need or invoking legal requirements for mandatory requests have not proved successful (Clark, Robinson, & Wicklegren, 1988). The present study suggests that research on the psychology of organ donation may be beneficial.

Second, the lawfulness of the present results is striking. That implies that people are not random or unpredictable in their decisions to donate organs. On the contrary, there are clear patterns that have unexpected and as yet unappreciated consequences. Looking for such patterns should be a goal in future research.

Third, the findings show that few people are opposed to donation; almost everyone will donate—if the circumstances are right. The reported reluctance of doctors and other medical personnel to contact next of kin may be based on a mistaken belief that there are large groups of people unwilling to think about or consider donation. In contrast, the present results suggest that most people are supportive of donation.

Fourth, the results for the four groups of organ donors form a clear and consistent pattern. The results across the groups, as in Figure 5, are quite orderly. The systematic pattern of these between-group differences suggests that a similar four-group breakdown may prove useful in other analyses of organ donation.

Finally, it is worth observing that the formal, structured IIT approach was able to produce important new insights into an applied area such as organ donation. This was true despite the fact that the methodology and research procedures used were less than optimal. Much of the prior behavior research on organ donation has lacked theory or structure (Shanteau, 1986). Consequently, the field suffers from an absence of accumulated knowledge and understanding. The use of techniques like IIT may provide a framework upon which to build such a knowledge base.

References

Anderson, N. H. (1981). *Foundations of information integration theory*. New York: Academic Press.

Anderson, N. H. (1982). *Methods of information integration theory*. New York: Academic Press.

Clark, M., Robinson, C., & Wicklegren, I. (1988, September 12). Interchangeable parts. *Newsweek*, pp. 61, 63.

Fellner, C. H., & Marshall, J. R. (1981). Kidney donors revisited. In J. P. Rushton & R. M. Sorrentino (Eds.), *Altruism and helping behavior*. Hillsdale, NJ: Erlbaum.

Manninen, D., & Evans, R. (1985). Public attitudes and behavior regarding organ donation. *Journal of the American Medical Association*, 253, 3111–3115.

McIntyre, P., Barnett, M. A., Harris, R. J., Shanteau, J., Skowronski, J. J., & Klassen, M. (1987). Psychological factors influencing decisions to donate organs. In M. Wallendorf & P. Anderson (Eds.), *Advances in consumer research* (Vol. 14). Provo, UT: Association for Consumer Research.

Shanteau, J. (1986). Psychological research on organ donation. In M. Venkatesan (Ed.), *Proceedings of the Fifth Annual Health Care Conference*. Snowbird, UT: Association for Health Care Research.

Wilms, G., Kiefer, S. W., Shanteau, J., & McIntyre, P. (1987). Knowledge and image of body organs: Impact on willingness to donate. In M. Wallendorf & P. Anderson (Eds.), *Advances in consumer research* (Vol. 14). Provo, UT: Association for Consumer Research.

PART TWO

SOCIAL PSYCHOLOGICAL AND SOCIOLOGICAL FACTORS

CHAPTER 7

THE SOCIAL DILEMMA OF ORGAN DONATION:
OPTING IN OR OPTING OUT—IS THAT THE QUESTION?

DICK J. HESSING

OVERVIEW

The legal regulation of organ donation after death may be based on either the permission of the donor (opting in) or the absence of any objection (opting out). In the opting-in system, *explantation* (the extraction of organs) is not allowed without the prior explicit permission of the deceased or of the next of kin. In the opting-out system, explantation is permitted unless prior objections have been made by the person concerned or, if he or she has not expressed an opinion, by the next of kin. This chapter reviews the research into people's willingness to donate organs conducted since 1970, with special emphasis on Dutch and American studies. Although this review is limited in this way, the results of the studies discussed here have a wider relevance. This research is of two types. The first is directed primarily toward what determines, in general, people's willingness to donate organs. The second type of research proceeds from the specific character of the opting-in system and views the possible shortage of donors as a social dilemma. Two strategies to solve this social dilemma are then discussed: an opting-out system and a required request system.

ORGAN DONATION IN THE NETHERLANDS

Donation of organs in the Netherlands follows the rules of an opting-in system, in which the donor card plays a central role. The number of donor card carriers in 1975 was 3% of the total population. In 1980 this figure increased to 6% and in 1982 to 9%. In 1987, an estimated 12% of the Dutch population had signed donor cards. However, in general only half the card signers regularly carry the donor card with them. At present, in only 6% of the cases in which the explantation of an organ is possible is a donor card carried and found. In order to have enough organs available to meet the need for transplantation, 50% of the Dutch population would have to carry such a card. (Elffers & Hessing, 1983). Given the slow increase in the number of donor card carriers however, this percentage will probably never be reached. It is obvious from several publications that a worldwide shortage of donors exists, especially in countries with an opting-in system (Cantaluppi, Scalamogna, & Ponticelli, 1984; Dukeminier, 1970; Dukeminier & Sanders, 1968; Oesterle, 1974; Stuart, 1984).

The number of kidney transplants in the Netherlands increases each year with a certain regularity: in 1966, 2 transplants; in 1971, 59; in 1976, 181; in 1981, 252; in 1987, 454. In spite of this increase, the number of people waiting for a kidney transplant continues to rise as well. In 1987, 1,164 patients were waiting for a donor organ, and the average waiting time had gone up to 3 years.

DETERMINANTS OF THE WILLINGNESS TO DONATE ORGANS

Only a few years after it became technically possible to transplant organs and tissues of deceased donors, the first publication appeared about research into people's willingness to donate their organs after death in an opting-out system. Cleveland (1975, 1976; Cleveland & Johnson, 1970) was the first to research differences in motivation and willingness between potential donors (donor card signers) and nonsigners. Nonsigners showed more fear of death and burial; they avoided acknowledging their own mortality and believed more in life after death than signers did. Signers mentioned the following as important motives for donation: helping someone who is ill, advancing medical science, and feeling that the body is useless after death. Those who were not signers did not wish their bodies to be mutilated because, among other reasons, they believed that an intact body would be necessary for reincarnation (Cleveland & Johnson, 1970). Comazzi and Invernizzi (1974) concluded that an important condition contributing to ones's willingness to donate, at a rational level, was one's ability to come to terms with the unconscious fear of mutilation of the body and loss of bodily integrity. Also, Pessemier, Bemmaor, and Hanssens (1977) established a positive correlation between willingness to part with organs after death and feelings of charity, and a negative correlation between worry about the body after death and life after death. Claxton's study (1974), however, showed there was no correlation whatsoever between fear of death and behavior. Claxton imputed this to the fact that the scale he used—the Death Anxiety Scale (Templer, 1970)—consisted of items too divergent to measure the single dimension of fear of death (e.g., fear of one's own death, fear of the death of others, and fear of the future).

Large-scale research efforts into what influences the donor card signers—knowledge about various forms of transplantation procedures used in removing organs after death and the card signing itself—usually provide the same findings. In spite of considerable knowledge of, and a predominantly positive attitude toward, organ transplantation and donation, the percentage of donor card signers is much lower than one would expect on the basis of that attitude (Dutch Kidney Foundation, 1975; Moores, Clark, Lewis, & Mallick, 1976; Transplantation Council of Southern California, 1975). In 1975, the Dutch Kidney Foundation commissioned a study of knowledge, attitudes, and behavior regarding organ donation in the Netherlands. Although more than 90% of the respondents were acquainted with kidney and heart transplants, and 77% were willing to part with a kidney after death, only 3% were donor cardholders. Seventy-five percent of the interviewees were willing, in their capacity as next of kin, to permit the extraction of their relatives' organs if the deceased had indicated no objections. This rose to 90% if there was a donor card. The individual's expressed desires would, therefore, be respected in nearly all cases.

Research in the United States by the Transplantation Council of Southern California (1975) showed a similar pattern: Eighty-eight percent of respondents were acquainted with the various forms of transplantation, 77% had a positive attitude toward this method of prolonging and maintaining life, and 44% actually considered donating parts of their bodies after death for transplantation purposes. In spite of this, only 1% of the respondents were donor cardholders.

The same discrepancy between attitude and behavior was found in a study conducted by Eurotransplant (an international cooperative effort in the field of organ transplantation) of a representative sample of the Dutch population (see Hessing, 1983). In this study, 99% of the respondents fully agreed with the statement "It is a beautiful thought that sick people can be helped, thanks to donors," but only 6% of the respondents were donor cardholders.

In 1983, the Gallup Organization, conducted two surveys in the United States: one for the National Heart Transplantation Study (Manninen, 1984) and the other for the National Kidney Foundation (Gallup, 1984). In the first survey, based on a national probability sample of 2,056 respondents, the results showed that 94% of the respondents had heard about organ transplantation, 69% had heard of or received information concerning organ donation, and 14% carried a donor card. Of those not carrying cards, nonsigners, 28% were willing to carry such a card (i.e., 24% of the total sample). Furthermore, 53% of all respondents indicated that they would be willing to donate organs of a deceased relative if they had to make the decision, which was more than the numbers of persons willing to donate their own organs (50% for their own kidneys and 40% for their own skin or their own whole body).

The second survey consisted of in-person interviews of a nationally representative sample of 1,574 persons. More of the respondents (20%) cited "I don't like the idea of somebody cutting me up after I die" than any other reason for not donating their kidneys after their death. Every other reason stated was mentioned by smaller percentages of the respondents. Furthermore, this reason proved to be the greatest differentiator between those more likely and less likely to want their own kidneys donated: 5% and 44%, respectively.

In these two studies, the main trends in the results do not differ greatly. The attitude of the interviewees toward organ transplantation and donation is predominantly positive. They consider donating organs and tissues after death an altruistic deed. The decision to fill in a donor card seems to be influenced especially by both the attitude toward death and the appreciation of the body after death. It is remarkable to observe that researchers sometimes fail to make the distinction between a compulsory removal system and an opting-out system when questioning respondents in a survey. In a Eurotransplant survey (Hessing, 1988b), the attitude toward an opting-out system was measured by the statement "In most European countries it is not necessary that a physician ask permission for the extirpation of organs after death for transplantation. The same situation should be effective in the Netherlands." In Manninen (1984), the respondents were asked, "Do you feel that doctors have the power to remove organs from people who have died recently but have not signed a donor card without consulting the next of kin?" In both studies the percentages of respondents who agreed with the statements or answered *yes* (26% and 7%, respectively) were taken to suggest that an opting-out system would not be popular with the public. The essential difference between an opting-out system and a compulsory removal system has been obscured in the measures. In an opting-out system, one can, during his or her life, state an objection against donation after death, whereas in a compulsory removal system, there is no room for such a possibility. If the question of an opting-out system had been phrased more precisely and more validly, then the reponses favoring the measure might have been substantially higher. In Hessing (1983), 40% of the total respondents were in favor of an opting-out system, with no differences between those in favor of and those against organ donation after death.

Overcast and Merrikin report that "while the Uniform Anatomical Gift Act was an attempt to address society's interest in cadavers and organs as limited valuable resources for transplantation and medical study, the existing data suggest that the UAGA has been less than an overwhelming success" (Overcast & Merrikin, 1984, p. 27).

It is outside the scope of this chapter to discuss in depth the ethical aspects of health care, such as the right to health care and the distribution of health care. Viewpoints on this topic range from a conditional right to health care depending upon existing material resources (Jonsen, 1984) to defending the distribution of health care on the basis of need for such care as the most relevant application of the concept of justice to health care (Outka, 1976). From Jonsen's point of view, an opting-in system seems the only adequate legal system, whereas Outka's definition makes a stronger case for an opting-out system, in which society's interest in harvesting enough organs for transplantation ensures that the need for such care can be met.[1]

ORGAN DONATION AS A SOCIAL DILEMMA

Various authors have pointed out that there are no fundamental legal or legal–ethical differences between the opting-in system and the opting-out system regarding the individual's right of self-determination (Dukeminier, 1970; Stuart, 1984).[2]

In an opting-out system, however, society serves as an interested party, which supports donation. If a society is to go on functioning, it needs a cooperative attitude on the part of its members. If members are not sufficiently cooperative, then the authorities' task is to promote or command cooperative behavior.

From a psychological point of view, there is indeed an important difference between the two systems. In an opting-in system, in which a person signs a donor card, donation is considered an altruistic deed. A person is required to take steps to show willingness to donate an organ after death to another person. The opting-out system, however, proceeds from the idea that it is normal to donate organs because one feels morally obliged to save another person's life in this way. Those who do not want to contribute to this cooperative solution to the organ shortage have to take action to indicate their objections.

In the opting-in system, those who do not express an opinion are considered nondonors; within the opting-out system, they are potential donors.[3] There is thus a discrepancy in the current opting-in system between, on the one hand, a predominantly positive attitude toward donation, and, on the other hand, the low percentage of donor cardholders. According to the most recent data, only 12% of the population in the Netherlands hold donor cards, although it should be at least 50% in order to guarantee a sufficient supply of organs. Estimates for the United States range from 2%–3% of all those who are willing to donate (Overcast, Evans, Bowen, Hoe, & Livak, 1984) to 13%–14% of the total population (Manninen, 1984; Gallup, 1984). Because of the shortage of donors, fewer people can

---

1. "Our own death is indeed unimaginable, and whenever we make that attempt to imagine it we can perceive that we really survive as spectators. Hence . . . at bottom no one believes in his death, or to put the same thing in another way, in the unconscious every one of us is convinced of his own immortality." (Freud, 1925, p. 304)

2. Compulsory removal of organs is a third possible legal system. It is quite different from the opting-out (i.e., presumed-consent) concept as it is understood in those European countries that have adopted an opting-out system. Because the author knows of no example where a compulsory removal system has been introduced or is under consideration (with the possible exception of Soviet bloc countries), this type of system will not be discussed here.

3. It has become common practice to require family consent even if a person has signed an organ donor card (Overcast et al., 1984). These authors cite a transplant coordinator who reported that out of 600 donors in the past 7 years, only 3 carried donor cards. In the Netherlands the same situation exists. Common practice seems to have declared the donor card version of the opting-in system more or less obsolete. It might also be argued that in such cases, an opting-out system, more than an opting-in system, guarantees the individual autonomy, because in an opting-out system, the individual's wishes cannot be overruled by the wishes of the next of kin.

be considered for donation. This means not only that patients die, but also, in the case of kidney patients, that costly and lengthy treatments are used while the patient waits for a transplant. These costs will have to be covered by all members of society through health insurance.

In his seminal book *The Logic of Collective Action: Public Goods and the Theory of Groups*, Olson (1965) pointed out that it is not rational—in an economic sense—for individual users of public goods to contribute voluntarily to the production of those public goods. The supply of organs for transplantation can be considered a public good. When a considerable number of people become aware of Olson's observation that they can profit from a public good without contributing to it, a social dilemma exists—the conflict between individual benefit, on the one hand, and cooperative dependency, on the other. As a result, the number of voluntary contributions decreases, which results in a shortage of the public good. Maximizing individual gain in a situation of outcome-interdependence thus results in a collective suboptimum and consequently also in an individual suboptimum.

A SOCIAL ORIENTATION MODEL FOR INDIVIDUAL BEHAVIOR IN SOCIAL DILEMMAS

The decision within an opting-in system to carry a donor card is a decision under uncertainty: The chance that one will ever be a postmortem organ donor is only 0.7% in the Netherlands (Hessing, 1988a). The two foundations of the neoclassical theory of rational behavior under uncertainty as described by Von Neumann and Morgenstern (1947)—the subjective expected utility theory and the game theory—have both found their counterparts in social psychology. The subjective expected utility theory was introduced in psychology by Edwards (1954) and constitutes the core of the theory of reasoned action (Ajzen & Fishbein, 1980; Fishbein & Ajzen, 1975). Game theory has become known in social psychology as the social motivation theory through the work of Luce and Raiffa (1957) and Griesinger and Livingston (1973).

Fishbein and Ajzen, in particular, have elaborated the utility principle in their theory of reasoned action. According to this theory, the choice of behavior alternatives can be explained by attitudes and social norms. In this theory, an attitude is an evaluative reaction to the advantages and disadvantages of a specific act. The norm is the subjective estimate of the likely reactions of friends and relatives with regard to the act.

The social motivation theory is an attempt to explain individual behavior in situations in which people—in a situation of outcome-interdependence—have to allocate costs or gains or both. Social decisions reached in a situation in which the results are decided by both one's own and others' choices can be influenced by different factors. One of the most important is the weight that someone attaches to certain outcomes for himself or herself and others. Griesinger and Livingston (1973) have drafted a taxonomy of decision behavior in self–other

Variable	Behavior Concerns No Self–Other Allocations	Behavior Concerns Self–Other Allocations
When behavior is public:		
Attitude	Influence	Influence
[a]Norm	No separate influence	No separate influence
Social orientation	No influence	
When behavior is private:		
Attitude	Influence	Influence
[b]Norm	No influence	No influence
Social orientation	No influence	Influence

Figure 1 A social orientation model: The influences of attitude, norm, and social orientation on individual behavior in a social context. Data are from Hessing and Elffers, 1987.
[a]Norm and attitude coincide.   [b]Norm and attitude do not coincide.

allocations in such situations. The most frequent strategies that are used are cooperation (maximizing joint outcome), individualism (maximizing one's own outcome), competition (maximizing one's own relative outcome), and altruism (maximizing the outcome of the other).

When the social motivation theory and the theory of reasoned action are combined in one theoretical model, a social orientation model results, as in Figure 1. This social orientation model is a metamodel, a summary of models that will be relevant in special cases, depending on (a) whether the behavior in question is public or private and (b) whether the behavior concerns self–other allocations. The model predicts when attitude, norm, and social orientation will have an independent influence on behavior (Hessing & Elffers, 1987).

SOCIAL ORIENTATIONS IN ORGAN DONATION

In an earlier study, (Hessing, 1983) I tried to find an explanation for the discrepancy between the attitude toward organ donation and the low number of donor cardholders. In this study, the social orientation model was used as a basis for the hypothesis that, in addition to attitudes, the altruistic social orientation would be needed to explain the variance in behavior in this social dilemma.[4]

In working out this social orientation model, I used Batson's theory (e.g., Batson, Duncan, Ackerman, Buckley, & Birch, 1981) on various motivations possibly underlying altruistic behavior ("empathic concern" and "personal distress") and Weyant's theory (1978) on costs and benefits as intermediating

4. It is unlikely that everybody will react in the same way to social dilemmas. In general terms, people have different preferences for the distribution of benefits among themselves and others. These preferences are called social motives or social orientations (Liebrand and van Run, 1985; McClintock, 1972).

variables between self-esteem and altruistic behavior. On the basis of these two theories, it was hypothesized that persons with positive self-esteem have little cause to show altruistic behavior to further improve their positive self-image. On the other hand, a positive self-image gives rise to less self-concern, which creates the possibility for more empathy (Staub, 1978). If persons with positive self-esteem decide to behave altruistically, it stems from an empathic concern for the well-being of someone in need of help. This empathic concern can be lightened only by decreasing the other's suffering.

For persons with negative self-esteem, there is all the more reason to behave altruistically because this behavior may improve self-esteem. The experience of personal distress, however—although caused by someone else's situation—leads to a greater focus on one's own feeling of discomfort. This may be remedied by both altruistic behavior and shifting attention to other, less unpleasant situations. The choice between helping or shifting attention is determined, as Weyant proved, by weighing the costs and benefits of altruistic behavior. The costs, in the case of donating organs, have a bearing on the fear of death, which is associated with removal of organs after death (Hessing & Elffers, 1986). The benefit is the possibility of improving one's self-esteem.

The resulting model contained, therefore, the following three predictors: (a) self-esteem as a proxy variable for an altruistic social orientation, (b) the attitude toward organ donation as the attitude toward the act, and (c) the costs related to the fear of death in the case of organ donation and to the consequences of donor card holding, respectively. The results of Hessing's 1983 research confirmed the model: fifty-one percent of the variance in behavior could be explained by these predictors. In a replication study (Elffers & Hessing, 1983), the model was compared to the Fishbein-Ajzen model by means of LISREL IV (Jöreskog & Sörböm, 1978). The social orientation model proved significantly more capable of reproducing the data. This led to the conclusion that the discrepancy between attitude and behavior in the case of organ donation can be explained by taking into account the influence of personality variables, which can hardly be changed because of their central position in the personality structure: the altruistic social orientation and fear of death. Also, at first sight, the other two determinants seem to be hard to change. The attitude toward organ donation is already predominantly positive, and donor card holding (inherent in the opting-in system) is associated with negative consequences.

Kruÿdenberg and Huismans (1986) compared this model with the original Fishbein-Ajzen model. Next to the intention to carry a donor card, the actual carrying of such a card was a central variable in their study. Although the intention to carry a donor card could be explained by the Fishbein-Ajzen variables attitude and norm, these variables were unable to explain the actual act of carrying such a card. This behavior, however, could be very satisfactorily explained by the variables of the social orientation model.

From a rather different perspective, more evidence can be found in Barnett, Klassen, McMinimy, and Schwarz (1987). These authors recently published the results of a study in the United States on the influence of different public service announcements on the willingness to donate organs. The results showed that the respondents reacted more positively to announcements that stressed the advantages for the self than to announcements that stressed the advantages for the other—the potential organ receiver. The authors concluded that

> [the] results of prior studies may reflect the tendency of individuals to report socially desirable (i.e., other-oriented) responses. Such biases may be expected to play a significant role in survey . . . studies that ask people about their willingness and motive to help. In contrast, an experimental manipulation of motives for helping (such as used here) may serve to "camouflage" the socially desirable response, especially in a between-subjects design wherein a direct comparison of the "good" and "bad" motives is not salient. . . . [P]eople's motives for helping (when not directly solicited) may often reflect egoistic rather than other-oriented concerns. Research on individuals' reluctance to donate organs . . . concluded that "a barrier to organ donation is the fear that to do so will diminish the self, even after death." Perhaps the self-oriented [public service announcement] was found to be an especially persuasive message precisely because it emphasized an enhancement, rather than a diminution, of the self. (p. 336)

SOLUTIONS TO THE SOCIAL DILEMMA OF ORGAN DONATION

The solution to this social dilemma can be found in two ways. First, one could change the cost–gains structure of this social dilemma by the introduction of an opting-out system. Or, second, one could direct the request for permission or no objection more specifically, for example, to the location where a donor's organs become available.

Ninety-nine percent of the Dutch interviewees think it is good that people can be helped by means of transplants (Hessing, 1983). However, the opting-in system in the Netherlands, and the donor card requirement, poses too many obstacles to potential donors to transform that attitude into actual behavior. From a legal–psychological viewpoint, it may be stated that the difference between the two legal systems lies in the fact that in the opting-in system, cooperative behavior is hindered because the citizen must conquer one or more inhibitions, whereas in the opting-out system, cooperative behavior is taken as the starting point. In this system there is no single difficulty or inhibition to be conquered for an individual citizen to convert a positive attitude toward donation into action. With the introduction of an opting-out system, the cost–gains structure of this social dilemma is fundamentally changed. An elegant and socially just solution is found for a lack of altruistic behavior that cannot be remedied by law. In this system both cooperative and defective behavior are sanctioned on an individual level. Those who want to be potential donors after death will be so automatically, without having to take action, and those who refuse to take part in the solution of this social dilemma will have to take action to make their objections known.

There are, however, two difficulties with this solution. First, the introduction of an opting-out system, at least in the Netherlands, is likely to meet strong political opposition (Hessing, 1988a). A second obstacle can be deduced from the low number of organs harvested for transplantation in European countries with an opting-out system, which gives little reason for optimism. From this example, it can be surmised that the bottleneck in the supply of organs for transplantation occurs not only among individuals but also substantially among hospitals. The conclusion must be that the introduction of an opting-out system is the obvious way for solving the social dilemma insofar as it concerns the population, but that such a change in the system does not guarantee a solution to the shortage of transplantable organs.

It seems, therefore, more effective to find the solution in a more selective quest for organs. In practice this is already being done (Hessing, 1988b). Because so few people carry a donor card, it is not worthwhile, in the case of a possible donation, to search for a possible donor card. Currently, therefore, the next of kin are approached directly and asked whether they have any objections to the explantation of organs. The only problem that remains is that not all hospitals have adopted such a policy. The solution, then, is the introduction of a required request system. This system was introduced in the United States and the first results show an increase in donated organs (Caplan, 1984; Clark, Robinson, & Wickelgren, 1988; Fellner, Thistlethwaite, & Stuart, 1986; Kayali, 1986).

References

Ajzen, I., & Fishbein, M. (1980). *Understanding attitudes and predicting social behavior.* Englewood Cliffs, NJ: Prentice-Hall.

Barnett, M. A., Klassen, M., McMinimy, V., & Schwarz, L. (1987). The role of self- and other-oriented motivation in the organ donation decision. *Advances in Consumer Research, 14,* 335–337.

Batson, C. D., Duncan, B. D., Ackerman, P., Buckley, T., & Birch, K. (1981). Is empathic emotion a source of altruistic motivation? *Journal of Personality and Social Psychology, 40,* 290–302.

Cantaluppi, A., Scalamogna, A., & Ponticelli, C. (1984). Legal aspects of organ procurement in different countries. *Transplantation Proceedings, 16,* 102–104.

Caplan, A. L. (1984). Ethical and policy issues in the procurement of cadaver organs for transplantation. *New England Journal of Medicine, 311,* 981–983.

Clark, M., Robinson, C., & Wickelgren, I. (1988, September 12). Interchangeable parts. *Newsweek, 7,* 45–46.

Claxton, R. N. (1974). *A study of attitude and "other variables" in the prediction of commitment behavior regarding human organ donation.* Memphis: George Peabody College for Teachers.

Cleveland, S. E. (1975). Personality characteristics, body image and social attitudes of organ transplant donors versus nondonors. *Psychosomatic Medicine, 37,* 319–330.

Cleveland, S. E. (1976). Jehovah's Witnesses and human tissue donation. *Journal of Clinical Psychology, 32,* 453–458.

Cleveland, S. E., & Johnson, D. L. (1970). Motivation and readiness of potential human tissue donors and nondonors, *Psychosomatic Medicine, 32,* 225–231.

Comazzi, A. M., & Invernizzi, G. (1974). Emotional problems in young students offering transplantation organs. *Socijalna Psihijatrija*, *2*, 305–309.

Dukeminier, J. (1970). Supplying organs for transplantation. *Michigan Law Review*, *68*, 811–866.

Dukeminier, J., & Sanders, D. (1968). Organ transplantation: A proposal for routine salvaging of cadaver organs. *New England Journal of Medicine*, *279*, 413–419.

Dutch Kidney Foundation. (1975). *Onderzoek inzake niertrans plantaties* [Study on kidney transplantations] (Rapport 0 5618). Amsterdam: Author. Unpublished report.

Edwards, W. (1954). Theory of decision making. *Psychological Bulletin*, *51*, 380–417.

Elffers, H., & Hessing, D. J. (1983). Development in models for attitude–behavior relations: The case of organ donation after death. In *Multivariate analysis in the social and behavioural sciences 1983* (Publication 272, pp. 117–140). Amsterdam: Stichting Interuniversitair Instituut voor Sociaal-Wetenschappelijk Onderzoek.

Fellner, S. K., Thistlethwaite, J. R., & Stuart, F. P. (1986). Kidney transplantation from unrelated living donors. *New England Journal of Medicine*, *315*, 713.

Fishbein, M., & Ajzen, I. (1975). *Belief, attitude, intention and behavior*. Reading, MA: Addison-Wesley.

Freud, S. (1925). Thoughts for the times on war and death. In *Collected Papers* (Vol. 4, p. 304) London: Imago.

Gallup Organization, Inc. (1984). Attitudes and opinions of the American public towards kidney donation (Executive summary). Report prepared for the National Kidney Foundation. In R. W. Evans, D. L. Manninen, T. D. Overcast, L. P. Garrison, Jr., J. Yagi, K. J. Merrikin, A. R. Jonsen, et al., *The National Heart Transplantation Study: Final Report. Vol. 2. The availability of donor organs.* (Chapter 17, Appendix A). Seattle, WA: Battelle Human Affairs Research Centers.

Griesinger, D. W., & Livingston, J. W. (1973). Toward a model of interpersonal motivation in experimental games. *Behavioral Science*, *18*, 173–188.

Hessing, D. J. (1983). *De onsterfelijkheid benaderd: Een onderzoek naar de bereidheid tot postmortale orgaandonatie* [An approach to immortality: A study of the willingness to donate organs after death]. Lisse, the Netherlands: Swets & Zeitlinger.

Hessing, D. J., (1988a). *De regels van het spel* [The rules of the game]. Arnhem, the Netherlands: Gouda Quint.

Hessing, D. J., (1988b). Psychologische aspecten van orgaandonatie [Psychological aspects of organ donation]. In J. E. M. Akveld, F. Th. de Charro, D. J. Hessing, G. Kootstra, & H. D. C. Roscam Abbing (Eds.), *Orgaandonatie, een kwestie van bereidheid* [Organ donation, a matter of willingness] (pp. 49–69). Delft, the Netherlands: Vermande.

Hessing, D. J., & Elffers, H. (1987). Attitude toward death, fear of being declared dead too soon, and the donation of organs after death. *Omega*, *17*, 117–128.

Jonsen, A.R. (1984). Ethical issues in macroallocation of cardiac transplant. In R. W. Evans, D. L. Manninen, T. D. Overcast, L. P. Garrison, Jr., J. Yagi, K. J. Merrikin, A. R. Jonsen, et al., *The National Heart Transplantation Study: Final Report. Vol. 4. Ethical dilemmas.* (Chapter 38, pp. 1–35). Seattle, WA: Battelle Human Affairs Research Centers.

Jöreskog, K. G., & Sörböm, D. (1978). LISREL IV: *Estimation of linear structural equation systems by maximum likelihood methods*. Chicago: National Educational Resources.

Kayali, L. F. (1986). Early data on the impact of required request. *Dialysis & Transplantation*, *15*, 460.

Kruydenberg, A. P., & Huismans, S. E. (1986). *Donorcodicil, ja of nee? Een onderzoek in opdracht van de Nierstichting* [Donor card, yes or no? A survey for the Kidney Foundation]. Amsterdam: Free University.

Liebrand, W. B. G., & van Run, G. J. (1985). The effects of social motives on behavior in social dilemmas in two cultures. *Journal of Experimental Social Psychology*, *21*, 86–102.

Luce, R. D., & Raiffa, H. (1957). *Games and decisions: Introduction and critical survey.* New York: Wiley.

Manninen, D. L. (1984). Potential organ donor availability: Results of an attitude survey. In R. W. Evans, D. L. Manninen, T. D. Overcast, L. P. Garrison, Jr., J. Yagi, K. J. Merrikin, A. R. Jonsen, et al., *The National Heart Transplantation Study: Final Report. Vol. 2. The availability of donor organs. (Chapter 17, pp. 1–29).* Seattle, WA: Battelle Human Affairs Research Centers.

McClintock, C. G. (1972). Social motivation—a set of propositions. *Behavioral Science, 17,* 438–454.

Moores, B., Clarke, G., Lewis, B. R., & Mallick, N. P. (1976). Public attitudes towards kidney transplantation. *British Medical Journal, 1,* 629–631.

Oesterle, D. (1974). The sale of human body parts. *Michigan Law Review, 72,* 1182–1264.

Olson, M. (1965). *The logic of collective action, public goods and the theory of groups.* Cambridge, MA: Harvard University Press.

Outka, G. (1976). Social justice and equal access to health care. In R. Veatch & R. Branson (Eds.), *Ethics and health policy* (pp. 79–98). Cambridge, MA: Ballinger.

Overcast, T. D., Evans, R. W., Bowen, L. E., Hoe M. M., & Livak, C. L. (1984). Problems in the identification of potential organ donors: Misconceptions and fallacies associated with donor cards. *Journal of the American Medical Association, 251,* 1559–1562.

Overcast, T. D., & Merrikin, K. J. (1984). Legal issues surrounding the donor. In R. W. Evans, D. L. Manninen, T. D. Overcast, L. P. Garrison, Jr., J. Yagi, K. J. Merrikin, A. R. Jonsen, et al., *The National Heart Transplantation Study: Final Report. Vol. 2. Legal issues.* (Chapter 33, pp. 1–88). Seattle, Washington: Battelle Human Affairs Research Centers.

Pessemier, E. A., Bemmaor, A. C., & Hanssens, D. M. (1977). Willingness to supply human parts: Some empirical results. *Journal of Consumer Research, 4,* 131–140.

Staub, E. (1978). *Positive social behavior and morality* (Vol. 1). New York: Academic Press.

Stuart, F. P. (1984). Need, supply, and legal issues related to organ transplantation in the United States. *Transplantation Proceedings, 16,* 87–94.

Templer, D. L. (1970). The construction and validation of a death anxiety scale. *Journal of General Psychology, 82,* 165–177.

Transplantation Council of Southern California, (1975). *Public opinion and attitudes about medical transplantation among Los Angeles County residents.* Los Angeles: Author.

Von Neumann, J., & Morgenstern, O. (1978). *Theory of games and economic behavior.* Princeton, NJ: Princeton University Press.

Weyant, J. M. (1978). Effects of mood states, costs and benefits of helping. *Journal of Personality and Social Psychology, 36,* 1169–1176.

CHAPTER 8

THE SOCIAL CONSTRUCTION OF ALTRUISM IN ORGAN DONATION

HELEN LEVINE BATTEN

The act of organ donation offers the researcher a dramatic opportunity to analyze a social event because it occurs on the boundary between life and death. It raises into high relief personal connections to society and the social cohesion of the society itself. It is an arena in which the social construction of reality (Berger & Luckman, 1966) occurs under extreme psychological and social pressure.

There has been limited national empirical research about the experiences and perceptions of families who donate the organs of their relatives. An important study of Minnesota donors and their families conducted in the early 1970s by Simmons, Klein, and Simmons (1977, see also Chapter 10, by E. Borgida et al. in this volume) focused primarily on the experiences of living related donors (living donors who give an organ to a relative) and the effects of organ donation on family dynamics. However, Fulton, Fulton, and Simmons (1977) reported results from a small sample of 14 Minnesota families of cadaveric donors. The researchers concluded that organ donation goes more smoothly when the hospital attends to the needs of the donor family, because "the family, gives the gift of the organ, and they expect information, gratitude, or recognition in return." While the study by Fulton et al. was helpful in identifying some of the sources of stress faced by the families of cadaveric donors, the small sample size precluded analysis of donation experiences for members of different social groups. As Pearlin and Aneshensel (1986) have noted, different families have different resources available to them. Collins (1981) has asserted that individuals with more resources are more likely to have increased control over social interaction. Sufficient resources should provide social support for families under stress and could enhance a more altruistic reconstruction of their motivation for donation.

This chapter focuses on the social construction of the donor family's account of organ donation. The main thesis is that families will explain their decision to donate a member's organ as altruistic when they receive sufficient social support during the donation period. The first set of hypotheses to be examined is that three variables will lead to a positive social construction of altruistic motivation for donation: (a) greater personal resources, (b) higher social support, and (c) positive evaluations of the donation experience. A second set of hypotheses predicts that reports of enhanced coping will be associated with altruistic accounts of donation motivation and will also be associated with these three variables; that is, where families have more resources, they will be likely to garner more social support and to report coping more effectively with the crisis of the death of the donor. A third set of hypotheses predicts that family members who report fewer personal and social resources will be more likely to report conflict about the donation of a relative's organs. These family members are also expected to be less likely to reconstruct their motivation for donation as altruistic and to find fewer coping benefits from the donation.

METHOD AND RESULTS

Sampling
In the spring of 1985, a 16-page questionnaire was mailed to a purposive sample of 396 families of cadaveric donors located in the Northeast, South, Midwest, and Southwest. The overall response rate was 61 percent; 242 families completed and returned questionnaires. In 22 cases, more than one family member filled out a questionnaire, raising the sample size to 264 donor family members.

The empirical data reported here offer additional information about the experiences of families of cadaveric donors. The analysis of results can provide the basis for a better understanding of social psychological factors influencing the expression of altruism. A list of variables used in the analysis appears in Table 1.

Altruism
Altruistic motivation was the first dependent variable studied. Durkheim (1933/1964), Gouldner (1973), and Titmuss (1971) associated altruism with social solidarity. Although it is difficult to test empirically the connection between social values and social cohesion, a study of the motivation for organ donation may clarify this relation. In the present analysis, altruism was expected to correlate with higher socioeconomic status, greater social support, and a positive evaluation of the donation experience.

I would like to thank Jeffrey M. Prottas, Dick Batten, and John B. Williamson for their advice and encouragement on earlier drafts of this chapter.

Table 1

VARIABLES IN THE ANALYSIS OF ITEMS FROM QUESTIONNAIRES TO
FAMILIES OF CADAVERIC DONORS ($N = 264$)

Variable	Mean	Standard deviation	Cronbach's alpha
1. "Our family believed our relative would have wanted to help someone else this way."[a]	0.792	0.407	
2. "Our family wanted to help someone else this way."[a]	0.803	0.398	
3. "We felt that functioning organs should not be wasted."[a]	0.644	0.480	
4. Altruism scale[b]	2.300	0.910	.65
5. "Do you feel organ donation has made coping with your loss any easier?"[c]	2.673	0.983	
6. Married respondents[d]	0.634	0.481	
7. Catholic respondents[d]	0.310	0.458	
8. Religiousness[e]	3.054	0.651	
9. Female respondents[d]	0.737	0.440	
10. Age in years	45.474	11.544	
11. Family first raised the option of donation.[d]	0.303	0.458	
12. When asked about organ donation, family member had accepted that relative would not live.[a]	0.725	0.433	
13. Number of people involved in decision to donate	2.936	1.013	
14. Relative was a multiorgan donor.[d]	0.723	0.448	
15. Intensive care unit (ICU) nurses were supportive of donor families.[f]	3.245	0.686	
16. Hospital doctors were supportive of donor families.[f]	3.128	0.687	
17. Organ procurement staff were helpful to donor families.[f]	3.166	0.657	
18. Hospital support scale[g]	3.175	0.529	.76
19. "I would consider donating my organs at the time of my death."[d]	0.861	0.367	
20. "If I had the decision to make again, I would choose to permit organ donation."[d]	0.963	0.189	

(table continues)

Table 1, continued

Variable	Mean	Standard deviation	Cronbach's alpha
21. Personal support scale[h]	0.896	0.263	.65
22. "The person who explained brain death did so clearly."[d]	0.816	0.382	
23. Conflict scale[h]	0.356	0.480	.76

Note. Mean values are substituted for missing values for values used in multivariate analyses. Where scales have been constructed, their components are listed above them and Cronbach's alpha reliability coefficients are also given.
[a]Range = 0–1 (1 = agree). [b]Range = 1–3 (3 = high). The altruism score was created by combining positive answers to items 1, 2, and 3. [c]Range = 1–4 (4 = much easier). [d]Range = 0–1 (1 = yes). [e]Range = 1–4 (4 = high). [f]Range = 1–4 (4 = strongly agree). [g]Range = 1–4 (4 = high). The hospital support score was created by combining positive answers to items 15, 16, and 17 and dividing by 4. [h]Range = 0–1 (1 = high).

The measures of altruistic motivation were based on self-reports of respondents. Self-reports of attitudes and perceptions of behavior may be distorted by the wish to give socially desirable responses or by lack of self-awareness. However, self-reports in mail surveys have been found to be useful indications of behavior or attitudes that are difficult for subjects to discuss or for researchers to observe (Williamson, Karp, Dalphin, & Gray, 1982).

To tap the respondents' concepts of altruism, they were asked how important it was for them to want to help someone else and not to waste functioning organs. Between 85% and 90% reported wanting to help others, and 75% felt organs should not be wasted. In the words of a mother whose 26-year-old son was fatally injured in an automobile accident: "My son was a generous and also a very healthy young man. . . . I knew if he could have been asked, he would have given himself so others could live."

Personal Resources

Three domains—personal resources, social support, and the donation evaluation—were hypothesized to influence the retrospective reconstruction of the motivation for donation as altruistic. Personal resources were hypothesized to be associated with reports of altruism. The six background characteristics used in this study to measure an individual's personal resources are (a) marital status, (b) income, (c) religious identification, (d) religiousness, (e) gender, and (f) age.

Demographic characteristics such as higher education and greater income levels are traditionally associated with socioeconomic status. However, educational level was not a good indicator of family socioeconomic status for this sample for two reasons. More women than men responded to the donor family survey, and this skews the relation between education and income; women survey respondents reported lower educational levels than men. Because married women's socioeconomic status was more likely to be tied to their husbands' educational level than their own, the women's educational status was an inaccurate indicator of the family's socioeconomic status. For these reasons, household income was a better measure of the donor family member's socioeconomic status.

Marital status and religious identification were considered indirect measures of socioeconomic status. Individuals who were married or who claimed identification having a religion with strong community affiliations, such as Catholicism, were more likely to have more personal resources. Those who indicated greater religiousness also were more likely to be involved in religious groups, which in turn leads to more social connections and therefore more opportunities to acquire social resources.

Age may be related to levels of socioeconomic status through the connection of age to income. Younger people may have lower incomes because they are just beginning their careers. In addition, those who are younger may have fewer social connections, because they have not yet established extensive social networks; this may also influence their socioeconomic status.

Gender may affect the accumulation of personal resources insofar as it affects income levels, especially for unmarried women. Single women who do not have a partner's income to draw upon may have a lower socioeconomic status. They may also be more isolated and therefore less integrated socially.

Social Support

Social support systems may also influence the expression of altruism. Social support for donor family members can come from within the family itself, but it can also come from the hospital. Donor family members interact with the institution of the hospital and other representatives of the health care system during and following the donation.

Family support was measured by five indicators: (a) the number of people involved in the decision to donate, (b) whether or not the family initiated the request for donation, (c) how well the family had accepted the fact that the donor was brain-dead at the time the donation was requested, (d) whether or not the family agreed to a multiorgan donation, and (e) whether they donated both the kidneys and the heart. The number of deciders was an indicator of the size of the respondent's support network at the time of donation. Pearlin and Aneshensel (1986) have commented that greater social resources ameliorate stress in a crisis. The assumption is that the more people there are involved who agree with the decision, the higher the respondent's degree of social support will be.

Where the respondent reported that the family raised the option of organ donation, and the family had accepted the donor's death when the subject of organ donation was broached, it was theorized that the family feels more in control of the donation events. The assumption is that better-integrated families will have sufficient resources to maintain some control over a situation that is otherwise desperate.

Two other factors that occur during the donation experience were thought to be indirect measures of the family support. Donor families must decide if they will donate only the kidneys or if they will donate other organs as well. It is suggested that the decision to agree to multiorgan donation is an indicator of clearer motivation to donate than is the decision to offer only kidneys. In addition, those who donated hearts as well as kidneys may feel they have made an important symbolic as well as actual contribution to society. This may also affect their reconstruction of their motivation as altruistic.

Finally, the respondent's assessment of strong hospital support was hypothesized to be associated with altruistic motivation. Support provided to the donor family by nurses, physicians, and the organ donor coordinator in the hospital may be a reflection of the family status. More cohesive families may report more positive interaction with hospital staff and higher levels of hospital support (Prottas, 1988).

The Evaluation of the Organ Donation Experience

Responding to the survey allowed family members to reconstruct a "story" of the donation experience. The social construction of reality proceeds in part through the objectification of an event and its externalization (Berger & Luckman, 1966). The retrospective reconstruction of the donation reality may be influenced by the socioeconomic status of the individual donor family member and the amount of social support that respondents experienced during the donation. Here it was predicted to influence reports of altruistic motivation for donation.

The evaluation of the donation experience may be deduced from respondents' answers to questions regarding (a) family members' personal support for donation, (b) whether or not they believed hospital or procurement staff had explained brain death clearly, and (c) whether family members had any problems with the donation experience. Personal support for donation was very high among respondents, as indicated by the fact that more than 85% expressed willingness to donate their own organs and 96% said they would choose to permit donation again. A personal support score was created by averaging the answers to these two questions (see Table 1, variables 19, 20, and 21).

Four out of five family members thought brain death had been explained clearly. There was a broader distribution along the conflict scale. More than 20% experienced high conflict, and more than 25% had some problems with the donation. However, nearly 40% expressed low conflict.

Conflict scores were measures derived from respondents' reports of problems in 16 areas of the donation experience. The four major problem areas were (a) being asked for donation too soon, (b) having to wait too long for the donation to be completed, (c) encountering billing problems after the donation, and (d) not receiving adequate feedback about what happened to the donated organs. Other problems mentioned by more than 10% of the respondents included in the conflict score were (e) difficulty in understanding that the donor was brain-dead, (f) cold, technical manner of staff presenting the concept of organ donation. (g) a lack of support from hospital staff, (h) uncertainty about scheduling the funeral, and

Table 2

COMPARISON OF CORRELATIONS WITH CONFLICT, ALTRUISM, AND
COPING

Domain	Conflict score	Altruism score	Coping
Socioeconomic variables			
Age	−.28**	.01	.06
Religiousness	−.17**	−.04	−.11
Female	.14*	.01	.05
Catholic	−.09	.11*	.05
Married	.08	−.05	−.12*
Income greater than $25,000	−.02	.16**	−.01
Social support variables			
Family support indicators			
Accepted death	−.24**	.14**	.17**
Family requested to donate	−.20**	.11*	.15**
Both heart and kidneys donated	.06	.09	.06
Number of deciders	.02	.12*	.10
Multiorgan donation	−.01	.15**	.14*
Hospital support score	−.36**	.21**	.32**
Donation evaluation variables			
Brain death clear	−.32**	.10	.28**
Personal support score	−.22**	.34**	.32**
Conflict score		−.16**	−.29**

*$p < .05$. **$p < .01$.

(i) lack of privacy. In addition, six problems reported by fewer than 10% of the
respondents were also included in the conflict score. These were (j) being asked
by too many people for donation, (k) feeling the staff acted too quickly in
declaring brain death, (l) feeling pressured by hospital staff to decide, (m) encountering conflicts with the funeral director, (n) having to wait too long before the
donation papers were signed, and (o) experiencing family disagreements. These
16 problem areas were used to create the conflict index.

Correlation analysis demonstrated that of the original 15 variables, 9 dis-
played statistically significant associations with the dependent variable, altruism
(see Table 2).

Multivariate Analysis of Predictors of Altruism

Because nine predictors were statistically related to altruism in the correlation
analysis, a regression was carried out regressing these variables on altruism (see
Table 3). Three of the nine variables were significant: the number of people
involved in the donation decision, the hospital support score, and the personal
support score. None of the indicators of personal resources retained their significance in predicting altruism.

Table 3

COMPARISON OF REGRESSIONS OF CONFLICT, ALTRUISM, AND COPING

	Beta weights		
Domain	Conflict	Altruism	Coping
Socioeconomic variables			
Income greater than $25,000	NE	.10	NE
Catholic	NE	.09	NE
Religiousness	−.12*	NE	.08
Married	NE	NE	−.12*
Female	.09	NE	NE
Age	−.23**	NE	NE
Social support variables			
Family support indicators			
Number of deciders	NE	.13*	NE
Family requested to donate	−.15**	.05	.08
Accepted death	−.10*	.08	.06
Multiorgan donation	NE	.03	.03
Both heart and kidneys donated	NE	NE	NE
Hospital support score	−.24**	.12*	.17**
Donation evaluation variables			
Personal support score	−.13*	.25**	.22**
Conflict score	NE	−.03	−.08
Brain death clear	−.20**	NE	.15**
R^2	.32**	.17**	.22*

Note. NE = Not entered.
*$p < .05$. **$p < .01$.

    The statistical tests weakly supported the first set of hypotheses relating personal resources, social support, and the evaluation of the donation experience to altruism. Through the multiple regression analysis, the number of significant predictors was reduced from nine to three variables: the number of people involved in the donation decision, the degree of hospital support the families received, and the personal support of the family members for organ donation. This finding demonstrated that support for altruism comes less from the personal realm and more from the social and attitudinal domains—it is influenced more by social than by personal factors.

    Theoretically, altruism and perceptions of coping are assumed to represent different realms of the donation experience. Altruism is a social value, and its prevalence is thought to reflect social cohesion. Coping perceptions are self-reports of the behavioral consequences of donation. In a sense, the coping benefit can be seen as the social exchange for organ donation. However, perceptions of altruistic motivation and coping showed a moderate statistical correlation (.38), indicating that altruism and coping perceptions may reinforce one another. Although it is difficult theoretically to determine which predicts which with the data at hand, they are both important aspects of the social construction of the experience of organ donation. Respondents' perceptions of coping as a consequence of the donation are investigated next.

Coping

As mentioned earlier, the second set of hypotheses to be tested in this chapter concerns the relation between personal resources, social support systems, evaluations of the donation experience, and perceived coping with the loss of a family member. Higher personal resources, greater social support, and positive evaluations of donation were expected to be positively and significantly associated with coping. In this section, the development of a measure of coping is discussed first. Next, significant predictors of coping are regressed on the coping variable to clarify the relation.

Measuring Coping

Some family members felt that donation gave a meaning to their grief. A mother of a 27-year-old son, victim of an automobile accident, compared the benefit she received from donating her son's organs to her sorrow that the organs of her son-in-law could not be donated after he was crushed to death in a work-related accident 15 months later: "I hope that all parents could be so fortunate. It has helped me to cope with my son's death and give it *some* meaning . . . . Our family talked about it again [when her son-in-law was killed] . . . feeling somewhat sorry that we couldn't do the same for B——."

The death of a relative—especially a young, previously healthy person who has been fatally injured in an automobile accident or suddenly struck down by an aneurysm—is a crisis, causing extreme stress. While the majority of respondents believed coping was made somewhat easier by the donation (61%), a substantial minority did not (39%). The indicator measuring coping was taken from a single item, which asks respondents if organ donation made coping with their loss any easier.

Correlations With Coping

Indicators from the three domains of personal resources, social support, and the donation evaluation were hypothesized to be associated with coping. Correlation analysis supported this hypothesis but revealed a somewhat different pattern of relation for coping than for altruism. Based on correlations, 9 variables of the 15 were significantly associated with coping: religiousness, marital status, whether the family asked for donation, whether the family had accepted their relative's death, whether they agreed to a multiorgan donation, hospital support, personal support, conflict, and the clarity of the brain death explanation.

Most of the variables differed from those found to be significantly correlated to altruism. From the first domain, income and Catholic affiliation were statistically related to altruism; in the coping analysis, neither of these was important. However, religiousness and unmarried status were correlated with coping. The relation with religiousness sustained the belief that this attribute is an important personal resource in coping with stress.

In the second domain (social support), there were also differences. The number of deciders did not correlate with coping, and the decision for multiorgan donation had a weaker relation with coping than with altruism.

The most striking differences were in the third domain (donation evaluation), where the clarity of the brain death explanation was moderately associated with coping, and the strength of the negative relation between coping and conflict was more pronounced than in the altruism correlation analysis.

Multivariate Analysis of Predictors of Coping

Using coping as the dependent variable, a multiple regression was conducted with variables in the three domains as predictors. The results of this analysis, depicted in Table 3, showed that 22% of the variance is explained when all nine variables are entered at once. However, only four variables remained statistically significant. These were: not being married, hospital support, personal support, and clarity of the brain death explanation. The conflict score was no longer significant when the variance explained by the other variables was taken into account.

Although the findings support the hypothesis about the relation between coping and measures of personal resources, social support, and evaluation of the donation experience, some of the results in Table 3 require further explanation. It was argued that being married was a measure of personal resources that was related to enhanced coping. An examination of marital status and coping revealed a negative association: Unmarried persons are more likely to report coping better than married people.

One interpretation is that coping with the loss of the role of mother or parent may be more difficult than coping with the loss of the role of spouse. Even though married individuals presumably have a partner to support them emotionally, they appeared to find the loss of a child most difficult to reconcile.

Another explanation may be that unmarried respondents were more likely to be formerly spouses of donors. While 63% of spouses of donors believed that their husband or wife felt positively about donation and felt they were doing what their relatives would have wished, only 36% of parents reported knowing about their child's attitude. Thus, spouses of donors faced less uncertainty in their decision than did parents.

When all the variables were entered, coping did not appear to be related to any indicators of family support in the social support domain. Instead, hospital support was significant. Coping with death through donation may be related to the recognition granted by the social system that receives the organs. Hospital support may indicate to the family member that the gift is being acknowledged at least by some of the professionals in the system. In this way, coping may be related to recognition of one's altruism.

The clarity of the brain death explanation may have helped to relieve family members of any guilt they might have felt in deciding to donate. Although their relative looked alive, the donor family member understood that he or she was dead. This awareness apparently reduced the psychological stress of donation for the family member.

The nonsignificance of the conflict score disconfirmed the hypothesis that high conflict reduces perceived coping. However, the conflict issue remains important theoretically and for its public policy implications. Theoretically, conflict may emerge because of the tension between family members' value of altruism and the norm of reciprocity that regulates most social exchanges (Gouldner, 1973). Public policymakers need to be aware of the potential for exploitation of some donor family members. The analyses showed some linkage between conflict, altruism, and coping. This relation is explored further in the following section.

Conflict

The family member's conflict score was negatively correlated with altruism ($-.16$) and coping ($-.29$). However, these relations were diminished and nonsignificant in the regression analyses of all independent variables. A closer examination of predictors of conflict scores may shed some light on this result.

As Table 2 demonstrates, there were three correlates of conflict from the first domain (personal resources). Younger people, family members without strong religious convictions, and women were most likely to report conflict from their organ donation experience. This pattern is very different from that found in the correlations between first domain variables and indicators of altruism or coping. Neither income level nor Catholic religious affiliation, the two correlates of altruism, was associated with conflict. Nor was being unmarried, the correlate of coping, related to conflict.

Among the indicators of family support, two were negatively associated with conflict scores: whether the family had initiated the request for donation and whether the family had accepted the death of the donor before being asked for donation. Family support appeared to be more important as a predictor of reported altruism than of conflict. Two out of the five indicators of family support were related to conflict, but four out of five correlated with altruism. Not surprisingly, the strongest predictor of conflict was negative hospital support.

The pattern of correlation is similar to the relation for coping, except the associations were all negative. Neither the number of deciders nor the decision to contribute more than kidneys, which showed some relation to coping perceptions, appeared to influence conflict reports.

The second strongest predictor of conflict ($-.32$ correlation) was found for clarity of the brain death explanation, a third domain variable. Compared to correlates of altruism and coping with third domain variables, personal support was less important in understanding conflict than was the family member's comprehension of the brain death explanation.

Multivariate Analysis of Predictors of Conflict

Regression of all eight variables representing the three domains accounted for more of the variance for conflict (32%) than for altruism (17%) or coping (22%). Sources of conflict appeared to come from all three domains when entered simultaneously. Table 3 displays these results.

Regression results lent support to the hypothesis that personal resources, social support, and donation evaluations separately and together affect the probability of encountering conflict in the donation experience. Three variables, each from a different domain, had the greatest effects on conflict: the hospital support, age, and the clarity of the brain death explanation.

Lack of support from hospital staff during the donation had the greatest effect on conflict reports. This finding underscores the importance of the family members' receiving recognition for their donation, as Fulton et al. (1977) noted. It also lends support to Jacobson's (1986) and Weiss's (1976) advocacy of the proper timing for social and emotional support of families in crisis. Younger people were most likely to feel the donation was problematic. Those without strong religious convictions also appeared to be more susceptible to problems with the donation than family members who may have more personal resources to draw upon during the crisis.

Personal support for donation was inversely related to conflict. This finding is difficult to interpret because it could be argued that problems during the donation may have affected reports of personal support when respondents completed the mail survey. In that case, personal reports would be dependent on conflict scores, rather than conflict scores being dependent on personal support. Unlike altruism and coping, personal support was not necessarily prior to conflict. In any event, personal support had less effect on conflict than the clarity of the brain death explanation. When family members remained confused about brain death, conflict was likely to be quite high.

DISCUSSION

A comparison of the full regression results of altruism, coping, and conflict reveals that no significant predictors from the socioeconomic domain are shared among the three dependent variables (see Table 3). While youth and lack of religiousness are predictive of conflict reports, only unmarried status is predictive of enhanced coping, and no socioeconomic indicators predict altruistic motivation.

Within the second domain, hospital support is predictive of all three dependent variables, inversely in the case of conflict. No significant indicators of family support appear for coping, and no significant predictors of family support are shared between altruism and conflict. The number of people involved in the decision to donate does predict altruism. Conflict is predicted if the family had not requested donation and had not accepted the fact that their relative was dead when they were asked for donation.

Personal support scores from the donation evaluation domain are shared predictors for all three dependent variables. Personal support is moderately predictive of altruism and coping, and it is weakly but inversely related to conflict. However, the clarity of the brain death evaluation is not associated with altruism, and lack of clarity is a stronger predictor of conflict than low personal support is. For coping, personal support is more predictive of enhanced coping than is a clear explanation of brain death.

Overall, the strongest predictors of altruism and coping come from personal support. The strongest sources of conflict—youth, low hospital support, and confusion about brain death—come from all three domains, and they are approximately equal in strength. Somewhat surprisingly, conflict is not significantly associated with reduced altruism. Although the negative relation between conflict and coping goes in the predicted direction, the absence of significance implies that other factors are more important to coping than a harmonious experience in organ donation. For example, problems encountered during the donation may be mitigated if, at the time of donation, families feel strong personal support for donation, believe hospital staff are generally supportive of them, and clearly understand that their relative is brain-dead.

The conflict analysis illuminated some of the sources of problems in the donation experience. Family members with fewer personal and social resources appear to have more trouble with donation. This finding lends support to the idea that the altruism of emotionally or socially poorer family members may not be adequately recognized.

The presence of hospital support contributes significantly to altruistic reconstructions of donation motivation and to the perception of higher coping among family members; the absence of hospital support is the strongest predictor of conflictual donation experiences. Although conflict does not have a significant effect on altruistic motivations, it bears an indirect relation through hospital support.

The private grief of donor family members takes on a public dimension when families are approached for donation by hospital personnel. The donation experience takes place within the overlapping institutions of the donor hospital and the organ procurement and transplantation system. The hospital is in a position to offer further social support to the family. However, the structural agenda of the hospital and that of the organ procurement and transplantation system may not always accord with that of the grieving family. As Collins (1981) asserted, individuals with greater emotional, cultural, and material resources have an advantage in directing social interaction to meet their needs. Families with greater personal and social resources are in a better position to influence their donation experience, whereas those with fewer resources may feel exploited by the system. In addition, when family support is weak, conflict is predictable.

Although altruism is more strongly influenced by indicators from the social support and donation experience domains, sources of conflict are also found in the domain of personal resources. The social construction of altruism is related to the social support the donor family receives during the donation, but the expression of altruism by more vulnerable donor families may be accompanied by more pain.

References

Berger, P. L., & Luckman, T. (1966). *The social construction of reality: A treatise in the sociology of knowledge.* Garden City, NY: Anchor Press.

Collins, R. (1981). The microfoundations of macrosociology. In *Sociology since midcentury: Essays in theory cumulation* (pp. 281–287).

Durkheim, E. (1964). *The division of labor in society* (G. Simpson, Trans.). New York: Free Press. (Original work published 1933)

Fulton, J., Fulton, R., & Simmons, R. (1977). The cadaver donor and the gift of life. In R. G. Simmons, S. D. Klein, & R. L. Simmons (Eds.), *Gift of life: The social and psychological impact of organ transplantation.* New York: Wiley.

Gouldner, A. (1973). *For sociology: Renewal and critique in sociology today.* New York: Basic Books.

Jacobson, D. (September, 1986). Types and time of social support. *Journal of Health and Social Behavior, 27,* 3.

Pearlin, L., & Aneshensel, C. (1986). Coping and social supports: Their functions and applications. In L. Aiken & D. Mechanic (Eds.), *Applications of social science to clinical medicine and health policy* (pp. 417–435). New Brunswick, NJ: Rutgers University Press.

Prottas, J. M. (1988). Shifting responsibilities in organ procurement: A plan for routine referral. *Journal of the American Medical Association, 260*(6), 832–833.

Simmons, R. G., Klein, S. D., & Simmons, R. L. (Eds.). (1977). *Gift of life: The social and psychological impact of organ transplantation.* New York: Wiley.

Titmuss, R. (1971). *The gift relationship: From human blood to social policy.* New York: Vintage Books.

Weiss, R. (1976). Transition states and other stressful situations. In G. Caplan & M. Killilea (Eds.), *Support systems and mutual help.* New York: Grune & Stratton.

Williamson, J., Karp, D., Dalphin, J., & Gray, P. (1982). *The research craft: An introduction to social research methods* (2nd ed., pp. 132–134). Boston: Little, Brown.

CHAPTER 9

PERCEPTIONS OF MEXICAN-AMERICANS AND ANGLO-AMERICANS REGARDING ORGAN DONATION ADVERTISEMENTS

PAT McINTYRE

RATIONALE FOR THE STUDY

Organ donation is an important social issue because thousands of people need donated organs in order to survive chronic diseases. These people depend on the goodwill of donors to provide them with life-sustaining organs after the potential donors die. However, there is a chronic shortage of donors and organs. To reduce the shortage, social advertising can be a valuable tool in informing the public about the need for organ donation and in allaying fears about the process. In this study, a social advertising approach was used to empirically examine the differences between Anglo-Americans and Mexican-Americans of comparable socioeconomic status in their response to organ donation public service announcements.

The Problem

Various studies have found that most Americans (93%–99%) have heard or read about organ donation (e.g., Gallup Organization, 1983). In addition, 70%–90% say they would be willing to donate their organs upon death. However, only 10%–20% have actually signed donor cards or the consent clause on the back of their driver's licenses. In 1983, only 3,000 organs were donated in the United States, although estimates show that 20,000 people could have donated organs.

Many studies have shown that people have some fears or concerns about organ donation that may prevent them from donating (Gallup Organization, 1983). In living donation, this fear is real. Donors may suffer pain from the operation, and living kidney donors, for example, may be at greater risk if the one remaining kidney becomes diseased. However, fear of donation after death is more difficult to explain. Prottas (1983) points out the topic of death as being almost taboo in our society. He states, "The primary cost of involvement in organ donation is confronting fear. One must admit and deal with one's own mortality" (p. 290).

The reasons mentioned above for not donating organs are very general. Some researchers have concentrated on specific psychological reasons why people do not donate. The Gallup poll (1983) found that 20% of sampled individuals stated that a very important reason for not donating was: "I never really thought about it" (p. iii). Another very important reason for not donating kidneys upon death for 20% of the sample was: "I don't like the idea of somebody cutting me up after I die" (p. iii). Prottas (1983) reported "that the most commonly expressed fear . . . is that agreeing to become a donor would negatively affect the treatment one receives in a hospital" (p. 290). Along these lines, McIntyre et al. (1987) found that the most important reason why people do not donate organs is their fear that a doctor would declare death prematurely for the sole purpose of obtaining their organs.

As mentioned previously, many people state that they are willing to donate organs upon death, but in reality they rarely do. This discrepancy between people's intentions to donate and their actual behavior is commonly found in the marketing and psychological literature. The problem, then, is how to bridge the gap between people's intentions and their actual behavior.

A Possible Solution

One of the ways to bridge the gap between intentions and behavior would be to use social advertising, which can be effective in at least five ways in regard to organ donation. First, social advertising is a way of reminding people about the need for organ donation. The advertisements can be played or shown at various times and with different themes to prevent people from forgetting.

Second, social advertising can be useful in transmitting information about organ donation, such as how many people are waiting for transplants, what kinds of organs can be donated, or how to become an organ donor.

Third, social advertising may be effective in directly addressing people's fears concerning organ donation. For example, as we stated earlier, some people are afraid to donate organs because they believe the doctor will declare them dead for the sole purpose of removing their organs (McIntyre et al., 1987). In this case, a social advertisement might tell them that, first, a team of doctors not connected with the patient would have to declare them dead. Those who fear mutilation and are concerned that they would not be able to have an open casket might be more likely to donate if they knew that organs are surgically removed and that the deceased could be viewed in an open casket.

Fourth, social advertisements may help convince people who are uncertain about organ donation to decide to donate their organs after death. Many researchers (e.g., J. J. Skowronski, chapter 11 in this volume; R. J. Harris et al., chapter 2 in this volume) report that a large percentage of people are uncertain about organ donation, whereas only a very small percentage are against organ donation. McIntyre et al. (1987) found that 32% of subjects stated that they would be willing to sign a donor card if asked to do so. Manninen and Evans (1985) believed that as many as 10% of persons unwilling to donate organs could be persuaded to do so. They also mentioned that only about 19% of the American population is truly unwilling to donate organs, whereas 53% are uncertain. To social advertisers this uncertainty means that a large percentage of the population might change their minds about organ donation.

Finally, social advertisements can be instrumental in getting families to talk with one another about organ donation. According to Prottas (1983), "People who act on the urging of the advertisement may act as opinion leaders on this issue in their families" (p. 289). For example, the same article reported that two surveys (one in Nashville and one in St. Louis) were taken of subjects both before and after a major public marketing effort. The percentage of people who discussed organ donation with their families changed considerably after the marketing efforts were completed.

It appears that social advertising can be effective in encouraging people to donate organs. If an advertisement is to be successful, however, it should convey a message that the viewer believes is relevant. Therefore, it is imperative for advertisements to stress information that is salient to the viewer.

The purposes of this study are to determine the source and type of message that would be most effective to different ethnic groups (i.e., Mexican-Americans and Anglos). Both the source and the type of message are extremely important in an advertisement and can influence its persuasiveness (Chaiken & Eagly, 1984).

The Effects of Ethnic Background

Ethnic background appears to be a major demographic variable related to organ donation. Several studies have investigated the differences between Whites and Blacks in their willingness to donate organs. These studies have found that Blacks are less likely than Whites to be signed donors, less likely to have favorable attitudes toward organ donation, and less likely to actually donate organs. Cleveland (1975) reported a 20% level of support for organ donation among Blacks in comparison to 67% support in the overall population. Prottas (1983) found that, although the Black population was around 29% in 8 cities studied, the Black donation rate was negligible, or not over 1%. He also found that transplant coordinators obtained permission from no more than 20% of the Blacks ap-

proached, whereas they usually obtained permission from 60% to 80% of the
White families approached.

Mexican-American Culture

The culture of interest in this study is the Hispanic culture, with an emphasis on
the Mexican-American subculture. "Hispanic," according to the Bureau of the
Census, refers to anyone who is of Spanish origin or whose native tongue is
Spanish. This includes Mexicans, Cubans, Puerto Ricans, and an "other" group
consisting of Latin-Americans. The largest subgroup of the Hispanic culture is
Mexican-Americans, who compose 60% of the total Hispanic population in the
United States (Cervantes, 1980). Puerto Ricans are second, followed by Cubans,
then "others."

Reasons for Selecting Mexican-Americans

Hispanics and Mexican-Americans in particular were chosen as the group of
interest because of four main reasons: First, the Hispanic population of the United
States is increasing at a rate almost seven times that of the general population
(Strategy Research Corporation, 1980). Because of this increase in birthrate,
Hispanics are expected to become the largest ethnic minority in the United States
by the end of the century. Further, the Hispanic population is so large that it
makes the United States the fifth largest Spanish-speaking country in the world
(Meyer, 1979). Almost one fourth (24.1%) of the Mexican-American families
have six or more people in them. This large number of Mexican-Americans
makes up a market that should not be ignored by organizations interested in
recruiting organ donors.

The second reason for selecting Mexican-Americans is their youthfulness.
The mean age of Hispanics is only 23.2 years compared to 31.3 for Whites and
24.9 years for Blacks (Petto, 1983). While 12% of the total United States
population is over 65 years of age, only 4% of the Hispanic community is in that
group (Segal & Sosa, 1983). The youthfulness of the Hispanic market may be
very appealing to organizations that wish to attract young organ donors. Young
people are preferred because they are usually in good health; thus, their organs
may help other persons for many years. In addition, in the United States young
people, irrespective of culture, are often involved in fatal accidents, and their
healthy organs can then be donated to others.

The third reason for selecting Mexican-Americans is their geographic concentration, which makes it easier to reach them with social advertisements.
Ninety percent of Mexican-Americans are from the states of the Southwest,
including Texas, California, Arizona, Colorado, and New Mexico. Texas has the
largest population of Mexican-Americans and includes cities such as El Paso and
San Antonio, which rank sixth and fourth, respectively in Mexican-American
population (Petto, 1983). This geographic concentration of Mexican-Americans

is very favorable for organizations that want to reach a majority of Mexican-Americans through regional advertising.

The final reason for selecting Mexican-Americans is the resistance of minorities to organ donation. It has been found that minorities in general are less likely to donate their organs than are Anglos (Prottas, 1983). Two studies done on Mexican-Americans and other Hispanics have found that they are more likely to refuse organ donation for their next of kin (Johnson et al., 1988; Perez, Matas, & Tellis, 1988).

Differences in Hispanics' Cultural Background

Formerly, it was commonly believed that Mexican-Americans were a homogeneous group, and all advertisements developed for one group of Hispanics were considered good for another group of Hispanics. According to Mendoza (1984), "social scientists assumed that all Mexican-Americans ate frijoles de la olla, spoke Spanish, and picked grapes for a living" (p. 61). But this assumption was incorrect. Cross-cultural researchers typically have compared random samples of Mexican-Americans with Anglo-Americans on some characteristics. Any differences that the researchers found between the groups were ascribed to "culture." However, the problem is that a sample of Mexican-Americans will incorporate people who differ on a variety of cultural characteristics, such as the ability to speak Spanish, their generational status, and ethnic identity. Since these often large in-group differences are not controlled for in the study, conclusions that were drawn about the effects of culture may be inaccurate. In addition, different advertisements may need to be developed to reach these various segments.

The Effects of Acculturation

There are two main ways in which the effects of culture can be investigated within the Mexican-American subgroup. One of these concerns the use of acculturation levels; the other way is through the use of ethnic labels. Acculturation refers to the process by which those new to a society adopt the attitudes, values, and behaviors of the host culture.

Level of acculturation is a psychological variable that has been measured in various ways. Generation may be the most important variable in predicting degree of acculturation (Clark, Kaufman, & Pierce 1976). Generation refers to the origin of one's parents and to one's place of birth. The first generation consists of people who are foreign born of foreign parents; the second generation consists of people who are native-born Americans but with one or both parents foreign born; the third or later generations consist of people who are native-born Americans with parents who also are native born. Because first- and second-generation children have been raised by foreign-born parents, the children may have absorbed the more traditional Mexican culture and therefore may be less acculturated to American society than third-generation children (Buriel, 1984).

These different acculturation levels may affect Mexican-Americans' willingness to donate organs and which advertisements they find appealing.

The Effect of Ethnic Labels

The second way to investigate the effects of culture is to segment subjects by their use of ethnic labels. An ethnic label is the term or name by which the people of a certain ethnic group prefer being called. There are many attitudinal differences between people who support various ethnic labels; for example, researchers (Fairchild & Cozens, 1981) have found differences between those who identify themselves as Chicanos and those who identify themselves as Mexican-Americans.

Montenegro (1976) found that Mexican-Americans were religious and attended church regularly, viewed men and women as having distinct roles within the family, saw hard work as being very important, and generally did not believe they were victims of discrimination. Chicanos, on the other hand, rejected hard work and competition, moved toward secularization, viewed both men and women as sharing roles within the family, and viewed themselves as being discriminated against. These results show that, because of different meanings associated with them, ethnic labels cannot be used interchangeably. Thus, ethnic labels can be used as a variable to segment Mexican-Americans on their willingness to donate organs and in the different advertisements that they find effective.

The Effect of Demographic Variables

In addition to considering levels of acculturation and the use of ethnic labels when conducting research on Mexican-Americans, it is important to consider demographic factors as well (Wallendorf & Reilly, 1983). There are two reasons: First, many researchers believe that cultural differences can be caused by noncultural factors such as socioeconomic status, for example, occupation and educational level. Penalosa (1968) believes that "Mexican middle-class persons are more like American middle-class persons in their general way of life and basic outlook than they are like lower-class persons from their own country" (p. 44). Socioeconomic class should therefore be considered in research on Mexican-Americans. Second, higher socioeconomic status is positively correlated with willingness to donate organs and may be a good segmentation variable to use in social advertising.

METHOD

Subjects

College students from the University of Texas at El Paso volunteered to participate in this study. There were 310 students, including 164 women (65 Anglo and 99 Mexican-Americans) and 117 men (51 Anglo and 66 Mexican-Americans). The remaining 29 students were from "other" ethnic backgrounds, including Chinese, Japanese, and Black students.

Materials

Students were asked to fill out a survey in English on organ donation and social advertising, rating the perceived impact of an advertisement using different sources and types of messages on a 7-point scale. The sources included a celebrity, a doctor, a religious leader, and an organ donor recipient. The types of messages included general background information, a religious message, an emotional message, and a message that addressed some fears people have about organ donation.

Procedure

Students were asked to complete the survey during their scheduled class period. Each student was offered extra credit for participating in the study. They were told to answer the questions honestly. After the survey was completed, the subjects were given a debriefing on the purpose of the study.

RESULTS

Perceived Impact of Source and Type of Message

Overall, both Mexican-Americans and Anglos chose an organ recipient as the best source of messages (mean = 19.0 out of a possible score of 28). The next highest source was a doctor (mean = 17.7), followed by a religious leader (mean = 16.2) and a celebrity (mean = 14).

Both Mexican-Americans and Anglo subjects also chose the informational message as having the most impact (mean = 17.9, out of a possible score of 28). The next highest message was an emotional message (mean = 17.6), followed by a message addressing fear (mean = 17.3) and a religious message (mean = 14.1).

Perceived Impact of Combination Source and Type of Message

The sources and types of messages were then combined to determine the combination with the most impact. The combination with the highest score was the organ recipient who gave an emotional message (mean = 5.4 out of a possible score of 7). The combination with the least impact was a celebrity with a religious message (mean = 2.9).

Table 1 gives the means for Mexican-Americans and Anglos of the various sources and types of messages. Most of the combinations were perceived similarly by the two groups, except for two. There was a significant difference between Mexican-Americans and Anglos in the impact of an organ recipient who gave a religious message; the mean of Mexican-Americans was significantly higher (mean = 4.1) than that of Anglos (mean = 3.6). In addition, there was also a significant difference between Mexican-Americans and Anglos rating religious leaders who gave an emotional message (4.3, for Hispanic, and 3.5, for Anglos).

Table 1

COMPARISON BETWEEN ANGLOS AND MEXICAN-AMERICANS OF
PERCEIVED IMPACT OF SOURCES AND MESSAGES

	Means	
Source and type of message	Anglo-Americans	Mexican-Americans
Celebrity, information	3.9	3.7
Celebrity, religious	2.8	3.0
Celebrity, emotional	3.8	3.7
Celebrity, addressing fear	3.6	3.5
Doctor, information	5.1	5.1
Doctor, religious	3.3	3.4
Doctor, emotional	4.7	4.4
Doctor, addressing fear	5.0	4.8
Religious leader, information	4.2	4.1
Religious leader, religious	4.1	4.3
Religious leader, emotional	3.8	4.3*
Religious leader, addressing fear	4.1	3.9
Organ recipient, information	5.2	5.0
Organ recipient, religious	3.6	4.1*
Organ recipient, emotional	5.4	5.4
Organ recipient, addressing fear	5.1	4.8

Note. The highest score possible was 7.
*Using an analysis of variance (ANOVA), these are significantly different at the .05 level.

Variables Within Cultures

There are three variables that may influence people within the same culture to respond differently to advertisements: income, ethnic label, and generation. Each was investigated in the study for the perceived impact of its source and type of message.

With regard to income, the first variable, there were two significant differences between those with a low family income (between $0 and $5,000 per year) and those with a higher income ($5,001 per year and up). Higher-income subjects were more likely to believe that an informational message from a celebrity (mean = 4.0) had more impact than did subjects of lower income level (mean = 3.6). In addition, higher-income subjects were more likely to believe that a message from a celebrity addressing fear (mean = 3.9) had more impact than did subjects with a lower income level (mean = 3.4). Because the highest possible score for each response was 7, however, neither group thought celebrities had a major impact.

In regard to ethnic term (Mexican-American or Chicano), the second variable, there were no significant differences in the students' opinions on the source and type of message.

Generation, the third variable, was the most important in producing differences in perceived impact of advertising. This variable (first, second, or third generation) showed significant differences in five different sources and types of messages, and it was close to significant for three other combinations (see Table 2). The first generation rated each of the combinations listed less favorably than the second or third generation did.

The source with the most perceived impact was the organ recipient, who was selected by both the Anglo and Mexican-Americans subjects. This is interesting because currently most organ donor advertisements use either a person needing an organ or a doctor to discuss organ donation. Although a person needing an organ was not one of the sources in this study, an organ recipient may be viewed even more positively by the public. This might be true because an advertisement focusing on a healthy person who was helped is seen as more positive than an advertisement with a sickly person who needs help. It would be valuable to investigate these two sources and determine which would have a greater impact.

The type of advertisement that had the most impact on Mexican-Americans and Anglo students was the information message, possibly because students are familiar with organ donation but do not know what organs can be donated and what the procedures for donating are. This is also relevant because most advertisements on organ donation use an emotional message.

Table 2

SIGNIFICANT DIFFERENCES IN PERCEIVED IMPACT OF ADVERTISING BY GENERATION

	Generations		
Source and type of message	First	Second	Third
Celebrity, information	3.0	3.8	3.8*
Celebrity, emotional	3.0	3.8	3.9*
Celebrity, addressing fear	3.0	3.6	3.7*
Doctor, addressing fear	4.3	4.8	5.0**
Religious leader, addressing fear	3.3	3.7	4.2*
Organ recipient, religious	3.4	4.1	3.7**
Organ recipient, addressing fear	4.5	4.6	5.1**
Organ recipient, emotional	4.8	5.5	5.5*

Note. The highest score possible was 7.
  *Using an analysis of variance (ANOVA), these are significant at the .05 level.
**Using an ANOVA, these are close to significant at the .065 level.

Concerning Mexican-Americans and Anglos, there were few differences in the source and type of message preferred, perhaps because all of the people in the sample were college students, which is a fairly homogeneous population. Even though college-educated people are more likely to donate organs than less educated people are, it is recommended that a more heterogeneous sample be used in future research.

There were two significant differences between Mexican-Americans and Anglos, both concerning either a religious leader or a religious message. These differences may have arisen because Mexican-Americans have more respect for religion and religious leaders in their lives than Anglos do as a group. Religion is tied closely to the Mexican-American culture.

Regarding variables within the Mexican-Americans culture, only two variables (income and generation) were significantly different. The use of ethnic labels was not significant.

The use of income (high vs. low) within the same culture proved to be significant in two cases. In both, celebrities were the source of the message. Although neither group thought celebrities had much impact, students from higher income levels gave a higher rating to celebrities, possibly either because these student are more likely to identify with celebrities or because they think others are likely to identify with celebrities.

The variable with the biggest impact was generation. The study showed that people of the first generation rated most sources and types of messages less favorably than people of the second and third generations did. First-generation students may be more suspicious of advertising in general, or they may have stronger negative beliefs about organ donation that cannot be changed with a simple advertisement. It may be best to concentrate on second and third-generation students for organ procurement.

In conclusion, more research on social advertisements concerning organ donation must be done to determine what constitutes the message with the most impact for each segment of the population in order to positively affect organ donation attitudes. The study in this report is a promising first step in obtaining the necessary information about Mexican-Americans and Anglos in order to persuade them to donate organs.

References

Buriel, R. (1984). Integration with traditional Mexican-American culture and sociocultural adjustment. In J. L. Martinez & R. Mendoza (Eds.), *Chicano psychology*. Orlando, FL: Academic Press.

Cervantes, F. (1980). The forgotten consumers: The Mexican-Americans. *Educators' Conference Proceedings* (pp. 180–183), Chicago: American Marketing Association.

Chaiken, S., & Eagly, A. (1984). Communication modality as a determinant of persuasion: The role of communicator salience. *Journal of Personality and Social Psychology, 45*, 241–256.

Clark, M., Kaufman, S., & Pierce, R. (1976). Explorations of acculturation: Toward a model of ethnic identity. *Human Organization*, *35*, 231–238.

Cleveland, S. (1975). Personality characteristics, body image and social attitudes of organ transplant donors versus nondonors. *Psychosomatic Medicine*, *37*, 313–319.

Fairchild, H., & Cozens, J. (1981). Chicano, Hispanic or Mexican-American: What's in a name? *Hispanic Journal of Behavioral Sciences*, *3*, 191–198.

Gallup Organization, Inc. (1983). *Attitudes and opinions of the American public toward kidney donation*. New York: National Kidney Foundation.

Johnson, L., Lum, C., Thompson, T., Wilson, J., Urdaneta, M., & Haris, R. (1988). Mexican-American and Anglo-American attitudes toward organ donation. *Transplantation Proceedings*, *20*(5), 822–823.

Manninen, D., & Evans, R. (1985). Public attitudes and behavior regarding organ donation. *The Journal of the American Medical Association*, *13*, 629–631.

McIntyre, P., Barnett, M., Harris, R., Shanteau, J., Skowronski, J., & Klassen, M. (1987). Psychological factors influencing decisions to donate organs. *Advances in Consumer Research*, *14*, 331–334.

Mendoza, R. (1984). Acculturation and sociocultural variability. In J. L. Martinez & R. Mendoza (Eds.), *Chicano Psychology*. Orlando FL: Academic Press.

Meyer, E. (1979). How to promote to Black and Hispanic consumers. *Advertising Age*, 54–55.

Montenegro, M. (1976). *Chicanos and Mexican-Americans: Ethnic self-identification and attitudinal differences*. San Francisco, CA: R and E Research Associates.

Penalosa, F. (1968). Mexican family roles. *Journal of Marriage and the Family*, *30*, 680–688.

Perez, L., Matas, A., & Tellis, V. (1988). Organ donation in three major U.S. cities by race/ethnicity. *Transplantation Proceedings*, *20*, 815.

Petto, A. (1983). The Hispanic market: A demographic and cultural profile. *Proceedings of the Third National Symposium on Hispanic Business and Economy in the 1980s* (pp. 136–148). Chicago: National Symposium on Hispanic Business and Economy.

Prottas, J. (1983). Encouraging altruism: Public attitudes and the marketing of organ donation. *Milbank Memorial Fund Quarterly. Health and Society*, *61*, 278–306.

Segal, M., & Sosa, L. (1983). Marketing to the Hispanic community. *California Management Review*, *26*, 120–134.

Strategy Research Corporation and the National Association of Spanish Broadcasters (1980). *The U.S. Hispanics—A market profile*. Miami, FL: Author.

Wallendorf, M., & Reilly, M. (1983). Ethnic migration, assimilation and consumption. *Journal of Consumer Research*, *10*, 292–302.

CHAPTER 10

THE MINNESOTA LIVING DONOR STUDIES:
IMPLICATIONS FOR ORGAN PROCUREMENT

EUGENE BORGIDA, ROBERTA G. SIMMONS, CYNTHIA CONNER,
KIRSTEN LOMBARD

With very few exceptions, most of the psychological research dealing with living kidney donation has focused on genetically related donors because such donation has been considered the alternative offering the highest survival rates for recipients (Brown & Sussman, 1982; Ewald et al., 1976; Fellner, 1976/77; Hirvas, Enckell, Kuhlbach, & Pasternack, 1980; Marshall & Fellner, 1977; Ringden, Friman, Lundgren, & Magnusson, 1978). This chapter presents a conceptual overview of research in progress at the University of Minnesota on the decision making of both genetically related and genetically unrelated, but emotionally linked, kidney donors. In this chapter the term *related donor* refers to living genetically related individuals (e.g., parents, siblings, adult children), and the term *unrelated donor* refers to living genetically unrelated individuals (e.g., spouses, friends). The first two sections of this chapter provide a brief review of previous research on genetically related and unrelated kidney donation. The third section of the chapter discusses some of the social psychological research questions addressed by the Minnesota living donor studies. The general presumption of the chapter is that the findings of living donor research can contribute to and enrich our understanding of the decision-making processes associated with cadaver donation and organ procurement.

GENETICALLY RELATED DONATION
Simmons and her colleagues have conducted programmatic and longitudinal research to evaluate the psychological reactions of genetically related donors and

their families (Kamstra-Hennen, Beebe, Strum, & Simmons, 1981; Simmons, 1983; Simmons & Anderson, 1982, 1985; Simmons, Klein, & Simmons, 1987). The psychological state of donors was compared to that of nondonors (family members who could have volunteered but did not do so) shortly after the transplant, with follow-up several years later. These findings suggested a much greater willingness to donate an organ than has been assumed by the lay or medical community (cf. chapter 6 by J. Shanteau & J. J. Skowronski in this volume). Donors were surprisingly willing to make this major sacrifice to save the life of a family member. Furthermore, the vast majority of those who did donate kidneys reported little or no ambivalence about the basic decision to do so. Concerns about surgery were not infrequent; however, in the majority of cases the decision to donate a kidney was described as instantaneous, made with no deliberation and usually with no later regret.

As late as 5–9 years posttransplant, the vast majority of donors indicated that they were without regret, and they were extremely happy that they had donated and that the recipient was alive and healthier. Feelings of increased personal closeness between donors and recipients were commonly reported after transplantation. Many donors received a great deal of family praise and gratitude both before and after surgery. Most interesting is the finding that donors' global self-esteem and level of happiness increased after the transplant as compared to control groups and nondonors; these improved feelings of well-being persisted at the 1-year follow-up and 5–9 years posttransplant (Simmons, 1983). Although most donors expressed positive attitudes, there was a small group of donors who were extremely ambivalent or regretful about their donation decision. Except for prior ambivalence, no one factor was found by Simmons and her colleagues to be highly predictive of later regret experienced by this subgroup.

Simmons and her colleagues also found some families for whom the donor search generated significant conflict and stress. Because of their reluctance or failure to volunteer, nondonors became the target of the hurt and anger of other family members. The nondonors' anger resulting from the perceived family pressure contributed to familial disturbances, although it was generally not directly expressed to the potential recipient. In all but a few cases, family stress and anger appeared to dissipate once the transplant was successfully performed. These tensions, however, could result in the long-term cost of lessened closeness to nondonors.

GENETICALLY UNRELATED DONATION

A review of the research literature reveals that relatively few studies have been conducted that directly address the psychological aspects involved in genetically unrelated living donation. Until recently, the lack of clear policies governing living unrelated donation has discouraged many transplant centers from tapping this source of kidneys. Transplant centers have also refrained from using unrelated living donors because of the complexity of the ethical considerations involved and the failure of such kidneys to function more successfully than cadaver kidneys

(Kountz, Perkins, Payne, & Belzer, 1970). Historically, there have been few cases in which unrelated donors were complete strangers to the recipient. One exception occurred almost two decades ago when prisoners who volunteered for transplantation were used as unrelated kidney donors (Crosbie, 1970). The practice was discontinued on the grounds that "the use of penal volunteers, however equitably handled in a local situation, would inevitably lead to abuse if accepted as a reasonable precedent and applied broadly" (Starzl, 1966, p. 76).

Sadler and colleagues (Sadler, Davison, Carroll, & Kountz, 1971) at the University of California–San Francisco were probably the first to study the psychiatric aspects of unrelated donation by using volunteers who were strangers to the recipient. In one year, three public appeals for volunteer donors generated calls from 200 persons; 22 became serious volunteers. Careful screening indicated that 17 of these were without psychological problems and that most were stable, middle-class citizens, married, with children. In only one donor case were social and psychological complications noted.

The use of living unrelated donors also failed to emerge as a viable option for many years due to the increased availability of dialysis and the belief that a well-matched cadaveric transplant was equally beneficial to the recipient without incurring any harm to a living donor (Levey, Hou, & Bush, 1986). More recently, however, attitudes toward living unrelated donation have begun to change as the shortage of cadaveric donors has persisted and as the medical technology of transplantation has improved. Transplant centers have increasingly begun to use donors who are genetically unrelated but emotionally linked to the patient (House & Thompson, 1988; Levenson & Olbrisch, 1987). Comparable or higher success rates than with cadaveric donors or living related donors have been reported (Kountz et al., 1970; Kumar, White, Samhan, & Abouna, 1987). Both the Council of the Transplantation Society and the American Society of Transplant Surgeons have recently approved the use of these "emotionally related" donors and have established relevant policy guidelines.

Quality of life studies reported by Simmons and her colleagues comparing alternative therapies for end-stage renal disease indicate that quality of life for successful transplant recipients significantly exceeds that of both continuous ambulatory peritoneal dialysis and in-center dialysis patients for nearly all variables tested, including physical, emotional, and social well-being. It is possible that as emotionally related donors are increasingly viewed as a viable alternative, friends and spouses may decide to donate a kidney rather than see another's quality of life compromised by extensive dialysis therapy in the event that a living related donor cannot be obtained, or during extensive waiting for an appropriate cadaver organ.

THE MINNESOTA UNRELATED LIVING DONOR PROJECT

At the University of Minnesota Hospitals' Transplant Center, both related and unrelated kidney transplants are now routinely conducted. Our research group has designed an extensive questionnaire on kidney donation that examines such psychological issues as quality of the donor–recipient relationship, beliefs about and attitudes toward donation, and decision-making processes involved with kidney donation. Some of the measures and scales used in previous research on genetically related donors and nondonors (Simmons et al., 1987) have been included. Our questionnaire is sent to all potential kidney donors (related and unrelated) who contact the university's transplant center and who express at least minimal interest in donating a kidney to a family member, spouse, or friend. By administering the questionnaire at a relatively early point in the donation process, we will be able to assess people who eventually go through with organ donation, as well as those potential donors who do not donate for whatever reasons. Thus, our data base includes survey data from genetically related and unrelated donors and nondonors. After the initial questionnaire is completed, clinical interviews are conducted and 1-year posttransplant questionnaires will be distributed. These survey data from unrelated donors, in combination with our clinical interviews of unrelated living kidney donors, will enable us to examine more closely the psychological processes accompanying the altruistic behavior of living kidney donation. In the remainder of this chapter we present an overview of three theoretical issues addressed by the Minnesota research on unrelated kidney donors: the quality of the donor–recipient relationship, donor decision-making processes, and the prediction of kidney donation. Implications for research on organ procurement are discussed in the concluding section of this chapter.

ASSESSING THE QUALITY OF THE DONOR–RECIPIENT RELATIONSHIP

One interesting but unexplored aspect of kidney donation involving unrelated donors is the quality of the donor–recipient relationship. Our research is somewhat unusual in the psychological literature because most studies focus on help providers who do not know the beneficiary of their altruism. In our study, the help provider knows the recipient quite well. Many of the unrelated donors are close friends of or married to the recipients of their kidneys. Previous research has typically characterized the donor–recipient relationship simply in terms of relationship *type*, such as mother–daughter, brother–sister, and so forth, rather than relationship *quality*. Our questionnaire contains items to examine three different social psychological models of relationship closeness, each of which we will test to see how well it predicts decision making and the final donation decision (see Clark & Reis, 1988, for a review of recent research on close relationships).

The first and most general model we use to characterize the donor–recipient relationship is the subjective closeness model (see Figure 1). This model is measured by two questions, each rated on a 7-point Likert scale, with the scores added to form a single index of subjective closeness. The two questions are "Relative to all your other relationships, how would you characterize your relationship with this person?" and "Relative to what you know about other people's close relationships, how would you characterize your relationship to this person?"

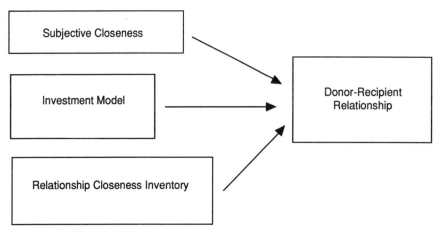

Figure 1 Theoretical models for assessing the quality of the donor–recipient relationship.

The second model is Rusbult's investment model (Rusbult, 1980, 1983). Rusbult breaks down the quality of the relationship into the components of rewards, costs, investment size, alternatives, satisfaction, and commitment. Commitment is then used to predict stay/leave behavior—whether a couple will break up or not. We have adapted Rusbult's measure for use in our research. The first four sections of items—covering rewards, costs, alternatives to the relationship, and investment size—begin with a definition of the term covered in that section. Donors are requested to answer both specific and global questions regarding these aspects of their relationships on a 9-point scale. Following this, donors are asked to answer several questions relating to satisfaction and commitment in their relationships as well. Rusbult has shown that the first five components can be used to predict commitment to the relationship, which we will then use to predict donation behavior.

The third model to be investigated is a behaviorally based conceptualization of closeness. Kelley and his colleagues theorize that behavioral interdependence between members of a dyad is the best indication of closeness in a relationship (Kelley et al., 1983). Interdependence can be characterized by high-impact interactions that are frequent and diverse, extending over a long period of time. The instrument we are using, devised at the University of Minnesota, called the Relationship Closeness Inventory, is based on this conceptualization (Berscheid, Snyder, & Omoto, 1988, 1989). It is broken down into three subscales: frequency, diversity, and strength of interaction. The items composing each of the three subscales are first used to tabulate a score on each scale independently and then added to form a single score, the closeness index. We will compare the predictive validity of this characterization of the donor–recipient relationship with the subjective closeness and investment models to determine which is the best indicator of kidney donation and the type of decision making involved.

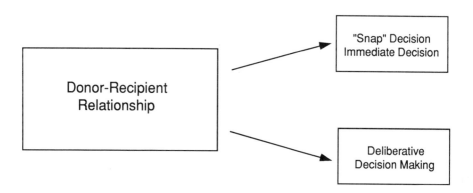

Figure 2 Types of decision making in living kidney donation.

Decision Making

We are also interested in examining more closely the decision-making processes of individuals who are deciding whether to donate a kidney. We are focusing on the extent to which decision making in this context is immediate or deliberative, as may be seen in Figure 2.

In immediate decision making, the decision is made quickly and without much thought or deliberation. The decision seems natural or the right thing to do. In deliberative decision making, the process may involve agonizing over the decision, systematically gathering information on which to base the decision, or talking to many people before making a decision. We have developed 21 statements characterizing people's decision making, and we ask donors to rate them on an 8-point scale. Some examples of each type are presented in Figure 3. We then ask them to rank-order the three statements that most closely describe their actual decision-making process. Our interest here is in determining whether an individual has made an immediate decision, one that may be based on strong feelings about the recipient, or has engaged in a more deliberative, cognitively controlled decision-making process in deciding to donate a kidney (Ajzen, 1985; Heckhausen & Beckmann, in press).

We generally expect that the level of closeness present in the donor-recipient relationship will be related to donor decision making (cf. Omoto, 1988). Donors whose relationships with the recipient are characterized by high closeness on these three models, for example, should report having made their decisions more quickly and with less thought than those who were low on closeness. We also expect that donors whose relationships are not characterized by high levels of closeness will be more deliberative and careful in their decision making, identifying processes similar to those captured by our deliberative statements in Figure 3.

Immediate Decision

When I first heard about the need for a kidney, I immediately volunteered.

Not at all close   1   2   3   4   5   6   7   8   Extremely close

I never thought it over; I automatically knew I would agree to donate.

Not at all close   1   2   3   4   5   6   7   8   Extremely close

I would say I made a "snap" decision in volunteering to donate a kidney to X.

Not at all close   1   2   3   4   5   6   7   8   Extremely close

It felt like an easy and natural choice to try to help another person.

Not at all close   1   2   3   4   5   6   7   8   Extremely close

Deliberative Decision

Once I heard that X needed a kidney I began to collect information about donating to help me make my decision.

Not at all close   1   2   3   4   5   6   7   8   Extremely close

I spent time thinking about the alternatives and weighing the pros and cons before I made a decision about donating a kidney to X.

Not at all close   1   2   3   4   5   6   7   8   Extremely close

I thought about all the possibilities and then made what I felt was the most logical and "best" choice.

Not at all close   1   2   3   4   5   6   7   8   Extremely close

I spent a lot of time thinking about whether to donate a kidney to X.

Not at all close   1   2   3   4   5   6   7   8   Extremely close

Figure 3 Examples of decision-making strategies.

Understanding and Predicting Kidney Donation

We are also examining the links between the donor–recipient relationship and actual donor behavior. To do this we will examine each of the three relationship models in the context of a more general theoretical framework—Ajzen's (1985) theory of planned behavior. The theory of planned behavior developed from the earlier theory of reasoned action (Ajzen, 1988; Ajzen & Fishbein, 1980). The latter is a model that has been successfully applied for the prediction of intention and behavior in such diverse areas as students' class attendance, problem drinking, weight loss, and blood donation (e.g., Schifter & Ajzen, 1985). According to this theory, the best predictor of a specific behavior is the *intention* to perform that behavior (see Figure 4). The stronger a person's intention concerning a specific behavior, the greater the likelihood that the behavior will actually be performed (Ajzen & Madden, 1986). The key assumption of this approach is that the behavior is under the person's volitional control.

The theory of reasoned action specifies that an individual's intention to perform a behavior is predicted by two independent components. One of the determinants of intention is *attitude toward the behavior*, which refers to an individual's favorable or unfavorable evaluation of the behavior. *Behavioral beliefs* (which are not shown in Figure 4) are defined as beliefs about the consequences of the behavior; these beliefs are weighted by their outcome evaluations. Behavioral beliefs are assumed to influence and predict an evaluative measure of attitude toward the behavior.

The other predictor of intention is a *subjective norm* component. Subjective norm is defined as the perceived pressure an individual feels to perform or not to

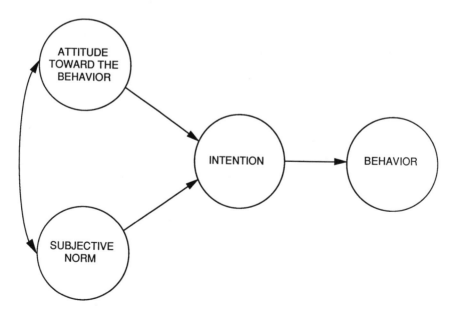

Figure 4 The theory of reasoned action.

perform the behavior. Although not shown in Figure 4, *normative beliefs* are considered the underlying determinants of the more general subjective norm measure. According to the theory of reasoned action, any other external variables, such as personality variables or demographics, are assumed to have only indirect effects on behavior.

Various assumptions must be met for the theory of reasoned action to adequately predict behavior from intention. For example, one of the assumptions, mentioned earlier, specifies that the behavior must be completely under the person's volitional control. However, many factors, both internal and external to the individual, can reduce a person's control over the intended behavior. If the performance of the behavior is contingent on the availability of certain resources or opportunities, performance then involves some degree of uncertainty. It appears that the theory of reasoned action cannot be generalized to those situations where this assumption is violated, that is, where there is *variation* in volitional control. In particular, behaviors that have addictive, habitual properties or behaviors that entail considerable affect tend to be behaviors for which there is variation in volitional control (Bentler & Speckart, 1979; Schlegel, d'Avernas, Zanna, & Manske, 1989).

By contrast, the theory of planned behavior, proposed by Ajzen (1985) as an extension of the theory of reasoned action, provides a predictive framework for a broader range of behaviors (see Figure 5). This model includes three components. The first two, as in the theory of reasoned action, are attitudinal and normative components. A third predictive component, unique to the theory of planned behavior, is referred to as *perceived behavioral control*. This third component represents an estimate of the perceived ease or difficulty of performing the specific behavior, based on a person's past experiences and anticipated obstacles. Beliefs about the presence or absence of necessary resources and opportunities are assumed to determine perceived behavioral control. By including an estimate of the individual's perceived control over the specific behavior, the theory of planned behavior allows for improved predictions of intentions and behavior.

Figure 5 also illustrates the two versions of Ajzen's theory of planned behavior. The first model includes a solid line, demonstrating the association between perceived behavioral control and intention that is not mediated by attitude or subjective norm. The second version of the theory of planned behavior includes the dotted line, representing the possibility of a direct causal link between perceived behavioral control and behavior. Perceived behavioral control may then influence and predict behavior indirectly through intentions and also directly as a measure of behavior. A direct link between perceived control and behavior is expected only if there is variation in volitional control over the target behavior.

In studying living unrelated kidney donors, we have applied the theory of planned behavior to examine and predict donation intentions and behavior. Because kidney donation is a behavioral domain in which there is variation in

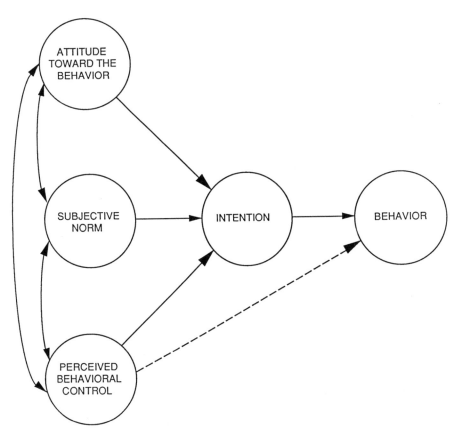

Figure 5 The theory of planned behavior.

volitional control (i.e., various factors beyond a person's control can affect the likelihood of donation), we expect that the inclusion of a measure of perceived behavioral control should increase the theory's predictive power. Not only is there variation in volitional control in this context, but kidney donation as an altruistic behavior probably is not as cognitively mediated as some other altruistic behaviors.

Figure 6 illustrates more specifically our use of the theory of planned behavior. As mentioned earlier, we have included and are testing various theoretical models of interpersonal closeness to measure the donor–recipient relationship. By including these measures of the donor–recipient relationship, we are hypothesizing that the inclusion of closeness in our model will improve prediction of the actual donation decision. Research on blood donation by Piliavin and her colleagues (Charng, Piliavin, & Callero, 1988) similarly found that prediction of donation was enhanced by adding the salience of role identity into a causal model based on the theory of planned behavior. We expect that, first, one's attitude toward donating a kidney will not be as cognitively mediated by behavioral intention as in other tests of the Ajzen model; second, a measure of relationship

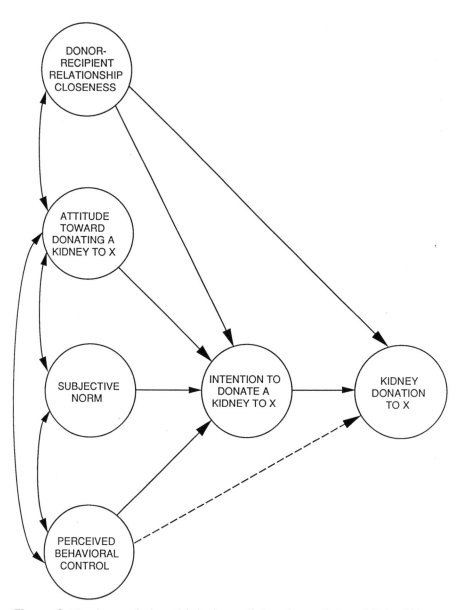

Figure 6 The theory of planned behavior applied to the prediction of living kidney donation.

closeness such as subjective closeness should have a direct rather than an indirect effect on actual behavioral choice; and third, perceived behavioral control should directly predict actual altruistic behavior.

CONCLUSIONS

Increased sophistication in surgical techniques and recent improvements in immunosuppressive procedures and histocompatibility matching have resulted in increased success rates for kidney transplant patients (Kountz et al., 1970). As these advances have enabled a greater variety of patients to become candidates for renal transplantation, the disparity between organ demand and supply has grown. Considerable effort has been directed toward increasing general awareness of the need for organs and increasing the number of people willing to donate organs in the event of their death (Perkins, 1987). Studies have found generally positive attitudes toward donation without, however, correspondingly high rates of signing organ donor cards (Cleveland, 1975; Corlett, 1985; Moores, Clarke, Lewis, & Mallick, 1976). The adverse psychological, economic, and medical consequences of a prolonged waiting period for an appropriate organ could be minimized by increasing the available supply of donor organs for transplantation (Perkins, 1987). An increase in living kidney donation may well have some impact, albeit modest, on the need for cadaveric donation and the anguish associated with currently lengthy waiting periods.

Living donor studies on the psychological nature of donor decision making generally represent a rather neglected data base for researchers who study cadaver organ procurement. Living donor research has investigated various social and psychological variables that may effectively differentiate individuals likely to donate from those less likely to donate. This research may eventually reveal informative similarities and differences between living donors and members of the public who are willing to donate their organs after death. For living kidney donors, donor–recipient closeness, as well as certain behavioral and normative beliefs about donation, may emerge as important predictors of donor decision making and donor behavior. Such findings would then support the appropriateness of applying the theory of planned behavior to the behavioral domain of donor card decision making. While there are obvious differences between these two decision-making contexts (e.g., stress levels, time frame), an understanding of individuals who are more likely to become living donors could be used to refine persuasive appeals about organ procurement for appropriate target groups within the general population. For example, living donors who have made a strong posttransplant adjustment may be effective advocates of organ donation to friends and acquaintances. Because friends and acquaintances represent credible and trustworthy persuasion sources, this form of information transmission of "social diffusion" based on interpersonal contacts (cf. Costanzo, Archer, Aronson, & Pettigrew, 1986; Darley & Beniger, 1981) could be incorporated into media-based persuasion campaigns. In addition, medical personnel could be encouraged to share their personal and professional experiences with the benefits and rewards of donation. Incorporating elements of this social diffusion approach into more traditional, media-based persuasion efforts may indeed bolster the effectiveness of current organ procurement campaigns.

References

Ajzen, I. (1985). From intentions to actions: A theory of planned behavior. In J. Kuhl & J. Beckman (Eds.), *Action-control: From cognition to behavior* (pp. 11–39). Heidelberg: Springer.

Ajzen, I. (1988). *Attitudes, personality, and behavior*. Chicago: Dorsey Press.

Ajzen, I., & Fishbein, M. (1980). *Understanding attitudes and predicting social behavior*. Englewood Cliffs, NJ: Prentice-Hall.

Ajzen, I., & Madden, T. J. (1986). Prediction of goal-directed behavior: Attitudes, intentions, and perceived behavioral control. *Journal of Experimental Social Psychology, 22*, 453–474.

Bentler, P. M., & Speckart, G. (1979). Models of attitude–behavior relations. *Psychological Review, 86*, 452–464.

Berscheid, E., Snyder, M., & Omoto, A. M. (1988). *The relationship closeness inventory: Assessing the closeness of interpersonal relationships*. Unpublished manuscript, University of Minnesota, Minneapolis, MN.

Berscheid, E., Snyder, M., & Omoto, A. M. (1989). Issues in studying close relationships: Conceptualizing and measuring closeness. In C. Hendrick (Ed.), *Review of personality and social psychology* (Vol. 10, pp. 63–91). Beverly Hills, CA: Sage.

Brown, C. J., & Sussman, M. (1982). A transplant donor follow-up study. *Dialysis & Transplantation, 11*, 897.

Charng, H., Piliavin, J. A., & Callero, P. L. (1988). Role identity and reasoned action in the prediction of repeated behavior. *Social Psychology Quarterly, 51*, 303–317.

Clark, M. S., & Reis, H. T. (1988). Interpersonal processes in close relationships. *Annual Review of Psychology, 39*, 609–672.

Cleveland, S. E. (1975). Changes in human tissue donor attitudes: 1969–1974. *Psychosomatic Medicine, 37*, 306–312.

Corlett, S. (1985). Public attitudes toward human organ donation. *Transplantation Proceedings, 17*(Suppl. 3), 103–110.

Costanzo, M., Archer, D., Aronson, E., & Pettigrew, T. (1986). Energy conservation behavior: The difficult path from information to action. *American Psychologist, 41*, 521–528.

Crosbie, S. (1970). The administrator in the organ replacement program. *Proceedings of the First International Symposium on Organ Transplantation in Human Beings*. Hanover, NH: Sandoz Pharmaceuticals.

Darley, J. M., & Beniger, J. R. (1981). Diffusion of energy-conserving innovations. *Journal of Social Issues, 2*, 150–171.

Ewald, J., Aurell, M., Brynger, H., Hanson, L. C. F., Nilson, A. E., Bucht, M., & Gelin, L. (1976). The living donor in renal transplantation: A study of physical and mental morbidity and functional aspects. *Scandinavian Journal of Nephrology, 38* (Suppl.), 59.

Fellner, C. H. (1976/77). Renal transplantation and the living donor: Decision and consequences. *Psychotherapy and Psychosomatics, 27*, 621.

Heckhausen, H., & Beckmann, J. (in press). Intentional action and action slips. *Psychological Review, 97*.

House, R. M., & Thompson, T. L. (1988). Psychiatric aspects of organ transplantation. *Journal of the American Medical Association, 260*, 535–539.

Hirvas, J., Enckell, M., Kuhlback, B., & Pasternack, A. (1980). Psychological and social problems encountered in active treatment of chronic uraemia III. Predictions of the living donor's psychological reaction. *Acta Medica Scandinavica*, 285–287.

Kamstra-Hennen, L., Beebe, J., Strum, S., & Simmons, R. G. (1981). Ethical evaluation of related donation: The donor after five years. *Transplantation Proceedings*, *13*, 60–61.

Kelley, H. H., Berscheid, E., Christiansen, A., Harvey, J. H., Huston, T. L., Levinger, G., McClintock, E., Peplau, L. A., & Peterson, D. R. (1983). *Close relationships.* New York: W. H. Freeman.

Kountz, S. L., Perkins, R. A., Payne, R., & Belzer, F. O. (1970). Kidney transplants using living unrelated donors. *Transplantation Proceedings*, *2*, 427–429.

Kumar, M. S. A., White, A. G., Samhan, M., & Abouna, G. M. (1987). Nonrelated living donors for renal transplantation. *Transplantation Proceedings*, *19*, 1516–1517.

Levenson, J. L., & Olbrisch, M. E. (1987). Shortage of donor organs and long waits: New sources of stress for transplant patients. *Psychosomatics*, *28*, 399–403.

Levey, A. S., Hou, S., & Bush, H. L., Jr. (1986). Kidney transplantation from unrelated living donors: Time to reclaim a discarded opportunity. *New England Journal of Medicine*, *314*, 914.

Marshall, J. R., & Fellner, C. H. (1977). Kidney donors revisited. *American Journal of Psychiatry*, *134*, 575.

Moores, B., Clarke, G., Lewis, B. R., & Mallick, N. P. (1976). Public attitudes towards kidney transplantation. *British Medical Journal*, *1*, 629–631.

Omoto, A. M. (1988). *Relationship involvement and closeness: Implications for the processing of relationship-relevant events.* Unpublished doctoral dissertation, University of Minnesota, Minneapolis, MN.

Perkins, K. A. (1987). The shortage of cadaver donor organs for transplantation: Can psychology help? *American Psychologist*, *42*, 921–930.

Ringden, O., Friman, L., Lundgren, G., & Magnusson, G. (1978). Complications and long-term renal function. *Transplantation*, *25*, 221.

Rusbult, C. E. (1980). Commitment and satisfaction in romantic association: A test of the investment model. *Journal of Experimental Social Psychology*, *16*, 172–186.

Rusbult, C. E. (1983). A longitudinal test of the investment model: The development (and deterioration) of satisfaction and commitment in heterosexual involvement. *Journal of Personality and Social Psychology*, *45*, 101–117.

Sadler, H. H., Davison, L., Carroll, C., & Kountz, S. L. (1971). The living, genetically unrelated, kidney donor. *Seminars in Psychiatry*, *3*(1), 86–101.

Schifter, D. B., & Ajzen, I. (1985). Intention, perceived control, and weight loss: An application of theory of planned behavior. *Journal of Personality and Social Psychology*, *49*, 843–851.

Schlegel, R. P., d'Avernas, J. R., Zanna, M. P., & Manske, S. R. (1989). *Problem drinking: A problem for the theory of reasoned action.* Unpublished manuscript, University of Waterloo, Ontario, Canada.

Simmons, R. G. (1983). Long-term reactions of renal recipients and donors. In N. B. Levy (Ed.), *Psychonephrology* (Vol. 2, pp. 275–287). New York: Plenum.

Simmons, R. G., & Anderson, C. R. (1982). Related donors and recipients five to nine years posttransplant. *Transplantation Proceedings*, *14*, 9–12.

Simmons, R. G., & Anderson, C. R. (1985). Social-psychological problems in living donor transplantation. *Transplant & Clinical Immunology*, *16*, 47.

Simmons, R. G., Klein, S. D., & Simmons, R. L. (1987). *Gift of life: The social and psychological impact of organ transplantation.* New York: Wiley Interscience.

Starzl, T. E. (1966). In discussion on J. E. Murray, Organ Transplantation: The practical possibilities. In G. E. W. Wolstenholme & M. O'Connor (Eds.), *Ethics in medical progress: With special reference to transplantation.* Ciba Foundation Symposium. Boston: Little, Brown.

CHAPTER 11

INCREASING THE NUMBER OF PEOPLE WHO AGREE TO DONATE ORGANS:
CAN PERSUASION WORK?

JOHN J. SKOWRONSKI

As a recent review by Perkins (1987) has noted, the success of organ transplantation technology has created a shortage of organs available for transplant. With further increases in the success rate of transplant operations, the shortage will become severe. Hence, one of the most important topics in organ donation research is to explore and evaluate ways of increasing the number of organ donors.

It is reasonable to speculate that the number of organ donors could be increased through the use of a promotional campaign that straightforwardly solicits donations. However, experience with social marketing campaigns indicates that promotional interventions have been most effective in bringing about behavioral change only when the audience is already favorable toward that change (Alcalay, 1983; Flay, 1985, 1987). A promotional campaign designed solely to induce people to engage in donation behaviors (such as signing a donor card) might cause behavior changes only in those who have not engaged in a donation-relevant behavior but who have a positive attitude toward donation. Further increases in organ donation behavior would depend on changing the attitudes of that portion of the population that continued to be unwilling to donate.

However, some might question whether a public service campaign designed to produce attitude change over the long term would yield any increase in donation behavior. For example, a number of studies have indicated that the American population consistently favors organ donation (e.g., see Prottas, 1983);

one might wonder whether further attempts at attitude change would be worthwhile in the face of this already overwhelming support. However, our research suggests that there are significant differences in attitudes between those who have signed a donor card and those who have not signed a donor card but who say that they would (McIntyre et al., 1987; Skowronski, 1987, 1988). Given these attitudinal differences and given that the proportion of the population that has signed donor cards is relatively small (less than 20% in our research), there may still be a considerable possibility of influencing donation behavior by changing donation-related attitudes.

This analysis suggests a number of potential research avenues for those interested in increasing the number of organ donors. In the short term, we need to know (a) how many people are potential targets of a campaign designed to induce donation-relevant behavior and (b) the methods that would effectively elicit those behaviors. In the long term, we need to know (a) the attitudes that affect why people do (or do not) donate organs, (b) whether those attitudes are changeable, and (c) the effective methods by which those attitudes may be changed.

In conjunction with colleagues, I have been engaged in a program of research aimed at answering some of these questions (McIntyre et al., 1987; Shanteau & Skowronski, chapter 6 in this volume; Skowronski, 1987, 1988). This previous research has focused primarily on the discovery of important attitudinal differences among various donor groups, but it has not been concerned with whether donation-related attitudes and behaviors are changeable, nor has it investigated the methods that would be efficacious in producing those changes. The issue of change is the prime focus of the research reported here.

More specifically, this chapter reports the results of an experiment using a "naturally occurring" persuasive presentation as the experimental manipulation. The presentation was both constructed and delivered by a representative of a local organ and tissue procurement organization.

The representative talked about organ donation to each of the sections of a general psychology class that was being taught on the campus in that term. Some students filled out a questionnaire dealing with organ donation issues before the presentation, whereas other students filled out the same questionnaire after the presentation. The impact of the presentation was evaluated by comparing the responses of the two groups.

Three issues related to attitude and behavior change were of primary interest. The first issue was whether the presentation would cause an increase in the number of people who signed or who would be willing to sign organ donor cards. The second issue was whether the presentation increased the willingness of

I thank Laura Davis for her help in analyzing the data for this study. I also wish to thank Lee Ann Welch, from Lifeline of Ohio Organ Procurement, for her cooperation in presenting the prodonation message.

Correspondence concerning this chapter should be addressed to John J. Skowronski, Ohio State University at Newark, Newark, Ohio 43055.

people to donate either their own organs or the organs of a deceased relative. The third issue was to assess the specific donation-related attitudes that were affected by the presentation (if any) and to relate those attitudinal changes to any changes in willingness to donate that might have occurred.

METHOD

Subjects

One hundred thirty students in general psychology classes at The Ohio State University at Newark participated in the study to partially fulfill course requirements. Sixty-eight subjects completed and returned the organ donor questionnaire before the prodonation presentation, and 62 subjects completed and returned the organ donor questionnaire after the prodonation presentation.

Organ Donation Questionnaire

An eight-page questionnaire was used as the dependent measure. This questionnaire had been fruitfully employed in prior research (see McIntyre et al., 1987; Skowronski, 1988). It includes the following sections (in order):

- ❑ Demographic information. These questions assessed general demographic information, such as age, gender, educational level, religious affiliation, and income.
- ❑ General donation knowledge/awareness/behavior. These questions assessed subjects' awareness of organ donation, their general knowledge about organ donor cards, and their knowledge about the organ donor card on the reverse side of their driver's license. One of these questions asked if subjects had signed the back of their driver's license, and a second question asked if subjects who had not would be willing to sign it. In addition, on a seven-point scale anchored by *strongly disagree* and *strongly agree*, subjects were asked to rate several general attitudinal statements dealing with organ donation.
- ❑ Personal motivation for donating. Using a seven-point scale anchored by *not important* and *extremely important*, subjects were asked to rate seven possible reasons for donating organs (e.g., altruism, increased self-esteem, helping the cause of science).
- ❑ Personal motivation for not donating. Using a seven-point scale anchored by *not important* and *extremely important*, subjects were asked to rate ten possible reasons for not donating organs (e.g., religion, fear of premature organ removal, desire to keep the body whole).
- ❑ Effects of transplantation use versus research use on willingness to donate organs. Using a seven-point scale anchored by *strongly disagree* and *strongly agree*, subjects indicated their agreement with six items of the form "If there were a _____percent chance that my

organs would be transplanted, I would agree to donate them." The instructions to the subjects made it clear that the other possible outcomes for the organs were disposal or medical research. Percentages ranged from 0% to 100%, in 20% increments.

☐ Next-of-kin issues. Using a seven-point scale anchored by *strongly disagree* and *strongly agree*, subjects were asked to rate their agreement with nine statements concerning the role of next of kin in organ donation. For example, one question asked how a doctor's request might affect the decision of next of kin to donate the organs of a deceased relative. Other questions asked whether a signed donor card should be overridden by next of kin or whether next of kin need to be consulted, given that the deceased signed a donor card.

☐ Religious factors. Using a seven-point scale anchored by *strongly disagree* and *strongly agree*, subjects rated their agreement with four statements assessing the impact of their religious community and their religious leader on the organ donation decision.

☐ Donor reimbursement attitudes. Using a seven-point scale anchored by *strongly disagree* and *strongly agree*, subjects rated their agreement with ten statements about the ethics and practicality of paying donors or next of kin for organs donated.

☐ Willingness to donate organs while alive. The questions in this section assessed, on an eleven-point scale anchored by *highly unwilling to donate* and *highly willing to donate*, people's willingness to donate, while alive, different specified organs to recipients who differed in their relationship to the donor. The relationships were brother/sister, son/daughter, friend, and stranger.

☐ Willingness to donate organs after death. This section assessed people's willingness to donate, after their death, different specified organs to either related or unrelated donors.

Prodonation Presentation

The prodonation message was presented in three parts. In the first part, subjects were shown a videotape that discussed the benefits of organ donation from the perspective of parents who decided to donate the organs of their deceased son. The second portion of the presentation consisted of a short talk that discussed some of the basic facts about medical aspects of organ donation (e.g., need for organs, procurement issues, number of operations performed, success rates, organ handling, lack of disfigurement); this discussion also covered the attitudes of major religious organizations toward organ donation and provided information about how to become an organ donor. The final portion of the presentation consisted of a question-and-answer session at which various issues, such as organ purchase and the legal force of donor cards, were discussed.

Procedure

To minimize demand characteristics that might occur as a result of the talk, strenuous efforts were undertaken to integrate both the experiment and the talk into the general routine of the psychology classes. In these classes it was typical for nonsensitive surveys to be placed in accessible locations along with drop boxes so that these surveys could be completed and returned at the subjects' convenience. The same procedure was used for the organ donation questionnaire, one of several surveys administered during the term. Before the presentation, a limited number of questionnaires were placed in the classroom used for all sections of general psychology. These prepresentation questionnaires were completed and returned at the subjects' convenience, from 1–4 weeks before the presentation.

All of the unused questionnaires were removed from the classroom 1 week before the presentation. Subjects who inquired about the availability of questionnaires in the 2-week period when no questionnaires were available (1 week before the presentation and 1 week after it) were told that no more surveys would be available until a new batch was photocopied. The need for, and a delay before, replenishment of survey material was not an infrequent occurrence with other survey materials delivered to the class. One week after the presentation, a new batch of organ donation questionnaires was put into the classroom. A separate group of subjects, at their convenience, completed and returned these questionnaires, from 1–3 weeks following the presentation.

A further attempt to minimize demand characteristics involved integrating the presentation into the "decision-making" unit of the class. The talk was presented as an example of the factors that affect decision making in a real-world problem.

Finally, it should be noted that the postpresentation questionnaires did not directly ask whether or not the respondent actually attended the talk. A question assessing this information was not included in order to reduce the demand characteristics that might have occurred if subjects connected the talk to the questionnaire. Although it is undoubtedly true that a few respondents in the postpresentation group did not hear the presentation, class attendance for the talk was quite good (87% of enrolled students were present); therefore, the number of people who did not hear the talk but completed posttalk questionnaires should be relatively small.

RESULTS

Because of space limitations, only the results of analyses that are pertinent to the effect of the prodonation presentation are presented below. Although a number of significant nonpresentation-related results were obtained in these analyses, these results are consistent with those of previous studies. See Skowronski (1988) and Shanteau and Skowronski (chapter 6 in this volume) for information about these other effects.

Table 1

COMPOSITION OF DIFFERENT DONOR GROUPS BEFORE AND
AFTER PRESENTATION

Time of completion of questionnaire	Donor		Positively disposed		Uncertain		Antidonation	
	n	%	n	%	n	%	n	%
Before presentation	6	8.8	10	14.7	36	52.9	16	23.5
After presentation	15	24.8	16	25.8	27	43.6	4	6.5

Changes in Behavior or Willingness To Donate Organs

Signing a Donor Card

As in past research (Skowronski, 1987, 1988), subjects were placed into one of four groups based on their responses to two questions. Subjects who indicated that they had signed an organ donor card were placed into the "donor" group. Subjects who indicated that they (a) had not signed their card but (b) would be willing to do so were placed into the "positively disposed" group. Subjects who indicated that they (a) had not signed their card and (b) weren't sure they would if asked to do so were placed in the "uncertain" group. Finally, subjects who indicated that they (a) had not signed their card and (b) would not sign it if asked to do so were placed into the "antidonation" group.

Table 1 shows the number of people who responded before and after the prodonation presentation, broken down by category of response. The data indicate that the prodonation presentation was effective: A higher proportion of those who responded after the presentation either signed their card or were willing to sign it than those who responded before the presentation. This difference was statistically reliable, $t(3) = 13.48, p < .01$.

Willingness To Donate Organs While Alive

These data were analyzed with a 4 (organ: kidney, skin, bone marrow, blood) × 4 (donor group: donor, positively disposed, uncertain, antidonation) × 4 (personal relationship: brother/sister, son/daughter, friend, stranger) × 2 (completion time: before presentation, after presentation) mixed analysis of variance.[1] This analysis produced only one statistically reliable effect involving the completion time variable, a significant Personal Relationship × Completion Time interac-

---

1. In evaluating the results of the analyses of variance reported in the present chapter, one should keep in mind that, because only four subjects were in the postpresentation/antidonor condition, the power of all statistical tests involving the interaction of the donor group and time of completion variables is quite low. This probably explains why there were no statistically reliable interactions between these two variables.

Table 2

EFFECT OF PERSONAL RELATIONSHIP TO RECIPIENT AND PRODONATION
PRESENTATION ON WILLINGNESS TO DONATE ORGANS WHILE ALIVE

Time of completion of questionnaire	Personal relationship to recipient			
	Son/ daughter	Brother/ sister	Friend	Stranger
Before presentation	9.06	8.65	6.50	4.15
After presentation	9.24	8.91	7.60	5.23

Note. 0 = *highly unwilling to donate*; 10 = *highly willing to donate.*

tion, $F(3, 366) = 4.48$, $p < .01$. The means for this interaction, presented in
Table 2, indicate that subjects in postpresentation groups were generally more
willing to donate organs than subjects in prepresentation groups, but the means
also indicate that the increase in willingness to donate organs was greater for
friends and strangers than for sons/daughters and brothers/sisters. This is probably because of a ceiling effect in the son/daughter and brother/sister conditions:
Subjects in the prepresentation condition indicated that they were quite willing to
donate to relatives, and consequently there was little room for increased willingness to donate as a result of the presentation.

Willingness To Donate Organs After Death
The data from this section of the questionnaire were analyzed with a 4 (donor
group: donor, positively disposed, uncertain, antidonation) × 2 (personal relationship: relative, stranger) × 2 (completion time: prepresentation, postpresentation) × 11 (organ: all, heart, lungs, kidneys, liver, pancreas, eyes, bones, skin,
brain tissue, sex organs) mixed analysis of variance. The only significant effect
involving the completion time variable was a Completion Time × Organ interaction, $F(10, 1200) = 2.02$, $p < .02$. The means for this interaction, presented
in Table 3, indicate that people who responded after the presentation were more
willing to donate organs than those who responded before the presentation, but
the increase in willingness was somewhat greater for the all-organs category, and
somewhat less for brain tissue and sex organs than for all the other organs.

Effects of the Relative Chances of Transplantation Versus
Research Use on Willingness To Donate Organs
The data in this section were analyzed with a 5 (transplant versus research
chances: 100%/0%, 80%/20%, 60%/40%, 40%/60%, 20%/80%, 0%/100%) ×
4 (donor group) × 2 (completion time) mixed analysis of variance. The results
of this analysis yielded no significant effects or interactions involving the completion time variable.

Table 3

EFFECT OF ORGAN DONATED AND PRODONATION PRESENTATION ON
WILLINGNESS TO DONATE ORGANS AFTER DEATH

	Time of questionnaire completion	
Organ to be donated	**Before presentation**	**After presentation**
All organs	4.73	7.15
Heart	5.88	7.65
Lungs	5.65	7.66
Kidneys	6.10	7.78
Liver	5.86	7.70
Pancreas	5.93	7.31
Eyes	5.30	7.92
Bones ·	5.23	7.07
Skin	5.69	7.61
Brain tissue	4.83	6.79
Sex organs	4.35	5.50

Note. $0 = $ *highly unwilling to donate*; $10 = $ *highly willing to donate*.

Next-of-Kin Issues: Willingness To Donate Organs of a Deceased Relative

Two items assessed people's agreement with statements asking about making a decision to donate the organs of a family member: "If a family member had just died and I did not know how he/she felt about organ donation, I would consider donating his/her organs," and "If a family member had just died and I did not know how he/she felt about organ donation, I would donate his/her organs." Responses to both questions were analyzed using a Donor Group (donor, positively disposed, undecided, anti donation) × Completion Time (prepresentation, postpresentation) between-subjects analysis of variance. Results indicated that the presentation had a significant effect on responses to both items. Subjects responding after the presentation expressed more agreement with both the first statement (prepresentation $M = 2.73$, postpresentation $M = 3.45$), $F(1, 119) = 3.47$, $p < .07$, and the second statement (prepresentation $M = 1.59$, postpresentation $M = 2.57$), $F(1, 121) = 5.00$, $p < .05$, than did subjects responding before the presentation. These changes apparently occurred in response to the videotaped portion of the presentation, which specifically dealt with the topic of donating the organs of a deceased relative.

Changes in Donation-Relevant Attitudes

Responses to all of the following attitude items were analyzed with a Donor Group (donor, positively disposed, undecided, antidonation) × Completion Time (prepresentation, postpresentation) between-subjects analysis of variance.

General Attitudes Toward Organ Donation

The presentation had a significant effect on responses to four of the six attitude statements in this section. Subjects responding after the presentation expressed more agreement with the following statements than did subjects responding before the presentation: "There are thousands of people in the United States who are waiting to receive donated organs" (prepresentation $M = 6.03$, postpresentation $M = 6.67$), $F(1, 121) = 4.35, p < .03$; "An organ donor has the potential to save many lives by donating all of his/her organs" (prepresentation $M = 5.64$, postpresentation $M = 6.19$), $F(1, 121) = 2.53, p < .12$; "The use of advertising would increase organ donation" (prepresentation $M = 4.95$, postpresentation $M = 5.54$), $F(1, 121) = 4.37, p < .05$; and "People would be more likely to donate their organs if they knew the organs would be used for transplant purposes than for medical research" (prepresentation $M = 5.15$, postpresentation $M = 5.79$), $F(1, 121) = 4.96, p < .05$. These results directly reflect the content of the presentation, which spent a good deal of time discussing the need for organs and discounting the possibility that donated organs would be used for research.

Personal Motivation for Donating Organs

The presentation had an effect on three of the seven attitude statements in this section. Subjects responding after the presentation rated the following items as more important reasons to donate than did subjects responding before the presentation: "To help others" (prepresentation $M = 6.19$, postpresentation $M = 6.59$), $F(1, 121) = 6.24, p < .05$; "To ensure my immortality (based on the belief that part of me will live on in another person after I am gone)" (prepresentation $M = 2.24$, postpresentation $M = 2.97$), $F(1, 121) = 6.50, p < .05$; and "Out of a sense of guilt (i.e., to attempt to undo some of the bad things I may have done while alive)" (prepresentation $M = 1.65$, postpresentation $M = 2.31$), $F(1, 121) = 6.50, p < .05$. It is unclear how the immortality item related to the presentation. The item about guilt may have been affected by the portion of the presentation that demonstrated the good that can come from transplantation.

Personal Motivation for Not Donating Organs

None of the eleven statements in this section were influenced by the presentation. Given that several of the statements in this section were directly addressed by the prodonation presentation (i.e., the possibility that organs would be discarded, use of the organs for medical research, disfigurement, and declaration of premature death), the lack of presentation-related effects in this section is somewhat surprising. Previous research (Skowronski, 1988) has indicated that these negative items might be important roadblocks to the donation decision; thus the failure of a relatively strong presentation to change these attitudes does not augur well for the prospects of a widespread promotional prodonation campaign.

Next-of-Kin Issues

The presentation had a significant effect on responses to three of the seven attitude statements in this section. Subjects responding after the presentation expressed lower levels of agreement with two of the statements than did subjects responding before the presentation: "If I indicated on the back of my driver's license or on my donor card that I want to donate my organs, my next of kin cannot legally refuse my wish" (prepresentation $M = 4.61$, postpresentation $M = 3.18$), $F(1, 119) = 18.80$, $p < .001$, and "If someone has signed a donor card, doctors should have the authority to remove organs without consulting the next of kin" (prepresentation $M = 3.29$, postpresentation $M = 3.08$), $F(1, 119) = 3.40$, $p < .07$. Subjects responding after the presentation expressed higher levels of agreement than did subjects responding before the presentation with the third statement: "Donating the organs of a loved one would bring me comfort and solace in my time of grief" (prepresentation $M = 2.73$, postpresentation $M = 3.85$), $F(1, 119) = 4.11$, $p < .05$. The presentation directly addressed the content of the first (legal refusal) and third (comfort) items, so these changes are apparently the direct result of the presentation. However, the effect of the presentation on items involving next of kin is paradoxical. Given that people generally seem to think that signing an organ donor card should have the force of a legal document (especially if the subject is the potential donor in question), it is somewhat surprising that the presentation should have caused people to decide to place even more power in the hands of the next of kin.

Religious Factors

The presentation had an effect on responses to only one of the four attitude statements in this section: "It is very important that my religious leader support my decision to donate" (prepresentation $M = 3.42$, postpresentation $M = 3.96$), $F(1, 106) = 3.99$, $p < .05$. It is unclear why the presentation should have affected this item and not other items (e.g., religious leader would support decision to donate) that were directly discussed in the presentation.

Donor Reimbursement Attitudes

The presentation had a significant effect on responses to four of the ten items in this section. Subjects responding after the presentation expressed more agreement with these statements than did subjects responding before the presentation: "The donation of organs should be done without financial compensation to the living donor" (prepresentation $M = 3.66$, postpresentation $M = 4.87$), $F(1, 119) = 11.17$, $p < .001$; "Living donors who might otherwise give organs for the purpose of helping others may decide not to donate if money was provided for their organs" (prepresentation $M = 2.78$, postpresentation $M = 3.42$), $F(1, 119)$ $= 4.24, p < .05$; "It is wrong for living donors to sell their own organs/tissues" (prepresentation $M = 3.54$, postpresentation $M = 4.13$), $F(1, 119) = 3.21, p <$ .08; and "It is wrong to buy human organs from a deceased donor (with the money going to the donor's family)" (prepresentation $M = 3.54$, postpresentation $M = 4.15$), $F(1, 119) = 5.22, p < .05$. It is obvious from the responses to these statements that the presentation, which discussed problems in procurement and the fact that some overseas buying is occurring, sensitized people to the organ purchase issue.

DISCUSSION

The experiment reported in this chapter evaluated the behavioral and attitudinal impact of a highly involving prodonation presentation. Three issues related to attitude and behavior change were of primary interest. The first issue was whether the presentation would cause an increase in the number of people who had signed an organ donor card or who reported a willingness to sign an organ donor card. The data from this study indicate that the presentation was somewhat effective in enhancing both card-signing behavior and willingness to sign a donor card. These results may encourage optimism about the prospects for increasing the number of organ donors in the short term. However, it should be noted that despite the fact that these changes were statistically reliable, the magnitude of the changes was not as great as one might hope. For example, before the presentation, 76.4% of the respondents were either uncertain or unwilling to sign donor cards. After the presentation, 50% of the respondents were uncertain or unwilling to sign donor cards. Thus, although there was a 26.4% decrease in the number of people in these two categories, a substantial portion of the postpresentation respondents were still not willing to sign a donor card.

The second issue of interest in this study was whether the prodonation presentation increased the stated willingness of people to donate either their own organs or the organs of a deceased relative. The results of the study indicated that the presentation was effective in increasing willingness to donate organs. However, the presentation was not overwhelmingly powerful in this regard. In the largest of the four donation groups, the uncertain group, the stated willingness to donate organs did increase as a result of the presentation. However, despite this change, in absolute terms these subjects expressed only modest support for donation. The best conclusion that can be drawn about the impact of the presentation on willingness to donate organs is much the same as that about the impact of the presentation on donor card signing: There was a positive effect, but it was probably not large enough to immediately affect donation behavior for most people.

Interestingly, the mean willingness to donate for subjects in the antidonation group was actually lower (although not significantly lower) in the postpresentation group than in the prepresentation group. If this effect proves to be reliable in future research, there are two interesting possible causes. This effect could reflect a self-selection bias: Those who were not extreme in their antidonation position could have been moved into the uncertain group by the presentation, leaving only the "hard-core" antidonation subjects behind. Alternatively, the presentation may have produced a reactance effect in the antidonation subjects, causing them to become even more unwilling to donate. One of the tasks of future researchers in this area should be to investigate the types of prodonation promotional campaigns that will not produce reactance in a portion of the population.

Of course, the significance of these "willingness to donate" data depends partly on the proposition that expressed willingness to behave in a certain way is actually a reasonable predictor of behavior. Although the use of self-reports of people's intentions as indicators of their ultimate behavior has frequently been questioned (see Wicker, 1969), recent research suggests that broadly based self-reports of behavioral intentions are often fairly good predictors of people's behavior (for a review, see Ajzen & Fishbein, 1980). Given the results reviewed by Ajzen and Fishbein, it is reasonable to expect that the changes in willingness reported by our subjects would ultimately be reflected in behavior changes.

The third issue of interest in this study was to assess the specific donation-related attitudes, if any, that were affected by the presentation and to relate those attitudinal changes to the changes that occurred in willingness to donate. Most of the specific attitudes that changed as a result of the presentation fell into one of five categories: an increased belief that organs are needed by others, an increased awareness of the help that can be given to others through organ donation, reinforcement of negative attitudes toward financially compensating donors or their families, an increased belief that donating organs can be psychologically beneficial to the donor or to the donor's family, and an increased awareness of the practical and legal issues involved when next of kin have to make a donation decision about a deceased relative.

Despite the fact that these attitudes were influenced by the presentation, there is no guarantee that these changes in attitude causally influenced the changes that occurred in willingness to donate organs. Prior research has demonstrated that some attitudes are more important to behaviors than other attitudes that are seemingly equally relevant (for example, see Fazio, Chen, McDonel, & Sherman, 1982).

However, some insight into the attitudes that may be important to the donation decision can be obtained by considering the results of the present study in conjunction with the results of previous research (Skowronski, 1988). In this earlier research, canonical discriminant analysis was used in an attempt to determine the relation between attitude items and donor group membership. One of the conclusions that can be drawn from canonical discriminant analysis is that items that have high canonical loadings are important to group membership. Hence, it seems reasonable to think that one might be able to affect group membership (i.e., willingness to engage in donation behavior) by changing attitudes with high loadings (i.e., high importance).

There were two items that both changed in response to the prodonation presentation in the present research and that received high loadings in this past research: (a) the item addressing the idea that donating the organs of a loved one could bring comfort in a time of grief and (b) the item stating that one reason to donate was to help others (the presentation certainly made people more aware of the fact that they could help and of the fact that others needed help). Although the data collected in this research certainly do not conclusively establish the causal impact of these attitudes on organ donation behavior, they do provide future researchers with ideas about the attitude changes that may lead to relatively swift behavior change.

The present research also points out areas in which a promotional program may encounter difficulties in inducing organ donation behavior. None of the items that related to people's unwillingness to donate organs were changed as a result of the prodonation presentation. Given that the presentation was a personal and involving one (in contrast to a relatively uninvolving mass-media presentation), and given that the presentation directly addressed many of these unwillingness items, this outcome is surprising. Further, because several unwillingness items may be important to the decision to be a donor (i.e., in past research they had high canonical discriminant loadings), this lack of change does not augur well for quickly increasing the number of potential organ donors. It seems reasonable to conclude that changing the attitudes that cause people to be unwilling to donate organs will probably be a slow process.

CONCLUSION

Based on this study, one's perception of the potential effectiveness of prodonation messages seems to depend on whether one is an optimist or a pessimist. The optimist might note that the prodonation message used in the present study did increase people's willingness to donate organs and did cause changes in some attitudes that are important to the donation decision. The pessimist, however, might point out that the amount of change was relatively small and that the presentation did not affect a number of important negative attitudes that influence the donation decision, despite the fact that these attitudes were directly addressed by the message.

Given the track record of many other similar public service campaigns, I am currently inclined to take a fairly pessimistic view of the situation. It seems clear that there are a few people who can, with relative ease, be persuaded to become organ donors. However, it also seems clear that the majority of the population will need a good deal of convincing before they finally make the decision to donate organs. The problem is that we do not yet know the methods or the specific concepts that would be the most potent producers of change, but it is hoped that this chapter makes a small contribution to our knowledge of these issues. Given the results of this research, however, I suspect that those of us who wish to use persuasive means to increase the number of organ donors have a long road ahead of us.

References

Ajzen, I., & Fishbein, M. (1980). *Understanding attitudes and predicting social behavior.* Englewood Cliffs, NJ: Prentice-Hall.

Alcalay, R. (1983). The impact of mass communication campaigns in the health field. *Social Science and Medicine, 17,* 87–94.

Fazio, R. H., Chen, J. M., McDonel, E. C., & Sherman, S. J. (1982). Attitude accessibility, attitude-behavior consistency, and the strength of the object-evaluation association. *Journal of Experimental Social Psychology, 18,* 339–357.

Flay, B. R. (1985). Psychosocial approaches to smoking cessation: A review of findings. *Health Psychology, 4,* 449–488.

Flay, B. R. (1987). Mass media and smoking cessation: A critical review. *American Journal of Public Health, 77,* 153–160.

McIntyre, P., Barnett, M. A., Harris, R. J., Shanteau, J., Skowronski, J. J., & Klassen, M. (1987). Psychological factors influencing decisions to donate organs. In M. Wallendorf & P. F. Anderson (Eds.), *Advances in Consumer Research* (Vol. 14, pp. 331–334). Denver: Association for Consumer Research.

Perkins, K. (1987). The shortage of cadaver donor organs for transplantation: Can psychology help? *American Psychologist, 42,* 921–930.

Prottas, J. (1983). Encouraging altruism: Public attitudes and the marketing of organ donation. *Health and Society, 61,* 278–306.

Skowronski, J. J. (1987, May). *Psychological factors influencing decisions to donate organs.* Paper presented at a meeting of the Midwestern Psychological Association, Chicago, IL.

Skowronski, J. J. (1988, April). *The psychology of organ donation: Toward an understanding of why people do (or don't) donate organs.* Paper presented at a meeting of the Midwestern Psychological Association, Chicago, IL.

Wicker, A. W. (1969). Attitudes versus actions: The relationship of verbal and overt behavioral responses to attitude objects. *Journal of Social Issues, 25,* 41–78.

PART THREE

CONCEPTUALIZATIONS AND IMPLICATIONS

CHAPTER 12

ME AND THEE VERSUS MINE AND THINE:
HOW PERCEPTIONS OF THE BODY INFLUENCE ORGAN DONATION AND TRANSPLANTATION

RUSSELL W. BELK

METAPHORS FOR THE HUMAN BODY

The confusion we may feel about whether our bodies are possessions or whether they are an essential part of us was described by William James:

> Our fame, our children, the works of our hands, may be as dear to us as our bodies are, and arouse the same feelings and the same acts of reprisal if attacked. And our bodies themselves, are they simply ours, or are they *us*? Certainly men have been ready to disown their very bodies and to regard them as mere vestures, or even as prisons of clay from which they should some day be glad to escape. (1890, p. 291)

Such ambivalence about whether our bodies *are* us or whether they are possessed by us suggests that we have not altogether accepted the Cartesian view of the body as a particular type of possession or thing—a machine. The model of the body as machine is one of several common metaphorical views of the body—each of which have significant implications for the psychology of organ donation and transplantation. If we regard our bodies as machines—at least as the sort of machines that we mass produce—then the idea of interchangeable parts provides a compelling extension of this metaphor that is quite compatible with the idea of organ transplantation. The body as machine metaphor has been dominant in 20th-century medicine (Johnson, 1987).

According to another metaphor, the body is a garden. The body is thought to be an object—but a natural or organic object rather than a synthetic object, as is implied by regarding the body as a machine. Extending this metaphor to organ transplantation is also fairly easy: Organs may be harvested and (im)planted (although not sown or grown).

A third metaphor for the body is the one alluded to by James: the body as self. If the body is seen as a central part of our identity, then a number of related beliefs and taboos may impede both the solicitation and successful transplantation of vital organs. Conversely, organ donation may be seen as a way to perpetuate the self—to gain a kind of immortality whereby a portion of the self extends to include organ recipients who continue to live after the donor's death. But whereas this metaphor may be advantageous for recruiting organ donors, it may present a problem for organ recipients who are adapting to their new organs. It is also a metaphor that medical professionals in the 20th century have tried to avoid and deconstruct (Young, 1989).

A fourth metaphorical view of the body is as a sacred vessel. From a religious perspective, if one believes that the body is a sacred temple of God, then mutilation of the body through organ donation may be considered as a sacrilege. There is also a nonreligious sense in which the body may be seen as sacred. According to this more worldly view, the body is a supreme source of hedonistic pleasure dependent only on its attractiveness (e.g., Featherstone, 1982). Whether or not the perception of the body as a temple is founded in religion, adherents have in common a reluctance to mar this perfect vessel, even after death.

The perceptions of self involved in each of these four common metaphorical views of the body have some important psychological implications for organ transplantation. The first two views of body as machine and body as garden are the most congenial to organ donation and transplantation, whereas the views of the body as self and as sacred each present certain difficulties or barriers to soliciting and transplanting organs. In this chapter, I provide a conceptual and theoretical apparatus and empirical evidence that may aid the reader in understanding these difficulties. It will also become evident that the metaphors of the body as self and the body as sacred are overlapping and mutually reinforcing.

ORGANS AS POSSESSIONS VERSUS ORGANS AS SELF

Sacred Self and Profane Commodities

A commodity is an object that has a use value and an exchange value. As Kopytoff (1986) observed,

> In contemporary Western thought, we take it more or less for granted that
> things—physical objects and rights to them—represent the natural universe
> of commodities. At the opposite pole we place people, who represent the
> natural universe of individuation and singularization. (p. 64)

Individuation and singularization are significant determinants of the sacred—that which is set apart, extraordinary, and powerful enough to produce feelings of ecstasy (Belk, Wallendorf, & Sherry, 1989). Whereas a commodity is mundane, ordinary, and profane, a sacred object is mysterious. It is revered. It is treated with the utmost respect.

A commodity can be exchanged for money with impunity and little emotion. But a sacred object is made profane by such a transaction (Appadurai, 1986). The sacred object can instead remain sacred, gain in its sacredness, or even become sacred by being given and received as a gift. If I buy a painting and decide tomorrow to sell it, no one is likely to be upset by these commodity transactions. But if my father who is an artist gives me a painting that he has done as a gift, it would be seen as a sacrilege if I should immediately decide to convert it into cash. To do so would be to alienate the inalienable (Gregory, 1980), to contaminate a sacred object of the self with money, to make profane the sacred.

In the case of body parts and organs, the 1790s French development of the anatomical–pathological model of disease spurred a great demand by physicians for cadaver dissection and for organs in particular. This led to the 1832 Anatomy Act in England, which allowed doctors the possession of the bodies of paupers for medical purposes (Laqueur, 1983). However, even this large supply could not meet the demand. The grave robberies depicted by Charles Dickens and Mary Shelley were real occurrences in this era when the bodies of the poor became market commodities. The horrific image of man created by Frankenstein is still sometimes used as an example of organ transplantation as a violation of the sacred body (Helman, 1988).

If the body is seen as sacred, it follows that the organs and tissues that constitute this physical body may also be seen as sacred. Using the body as a warehouse of parts threatens a key aspect of sacredness: the mystery of the body (Grange, 1985). When the cash crop, organ-farming practices of a fictional hospital were depicted in the movie *Coma*, Boston had no organ donors for hospitals for 43 days (Revkin, 1988). As an example of how organ donation can easily threaten to cross the line of commercialization, Fulton, Fulton, and Simmons (1977) reported that

> the brother of a cadaver–patient also objected to what he felt was the commercialization of the physician's approach to obtaining his brother's body-parts: To him it seemed "almost like stripping a car." (p. 361).

The U.S. Organ Procurement and Transplantation Act, passed in 1984, expressly stipulates that organs may not be treated as commodities and must instead by regarded as gifts. Prior to the passage of the act, one potential donor wanted to sell one of his kidneys to finance his way through graduate school, and entrepreneurs offered to act as brokers and put organ buyers and sellers together (Thukral & Cummins, 1987). Although some European countries, unlike the United States, have a policy of implied consent for cadaver organ donation, they too forbid organ donation for money and instead regard donating organs as a societal good.

Sacredness is used here in a way that may, but does not necessarily, involve formal religion. It might be expected that, in addition to public policy, religion is another guardian of the sacred status of the body; however, this is only partly true. Haney (1973) suggested that there are no theological barriers to cadaver organ donation. This is also only partly true. Judaism has been somewhat ambivalent about organ donation, and Islam opposes the removal (but not receipt) of cadaver organs. Buddhism actually encourages the donation of eyes so that the light can be passed on (Thukral & Cummins, 1987). Otherwise, the position of organized religions is currently neither to preserve the sacred body nor to encourage its exploitation. Uniformly, religious cremation, burial, and funeral rituals provide sacred rites and help console survivors. Although it is conceivable that organ removal might impede the effectiveness of these rituals, there is no evidence of such a concern among the major world religions, except Islam.

It is clear that the sacredness of the body and its organs is preserved when organs are removed from the legal category of purely private property. We have instead a "quasi-property" right to bodies—our own and those of our next of kin (Ramsey, 1970). The body cannot be used as security for debt payment, it must be disposed of in certain ways, and it can be the subject of a mandatory autopsy only under certain circumstances. The intent of these legal provisions is to ensure the sanctity of the body. "Proper respect for the body is irremovably a part of respect for the sanctity of the life of all flesh," says one expert in medical ethics (Ramsey, 1970, p. 208).

Thus, even when the body and its organs are considered to be possessions, medical, religious, and legal perspectives aim to ensure that our bodies remain sacred possessions rather than profane commodities. There is some evidence that the more sacred body parts are, the less likely they are to be donated to others. Wilms, Kiefer, Shanteau, and McIntyre (1987) found that people were less willing to donate organs that they understood less well and perceived as more sacred, emotional, and mysterious. The sacred–profane distinction is one important determinant of our regard for vital organs, but there is another important construct involved.

Organs as Part of the Extended Self

The extended self encompasses those tangible objects that are also seen as part of our identities (Belk, 1988a). Those tangible objects include our personal possessions, certain other people, our property and territory, and most important, our bodies and body parts. Philosophical debates concerning the degree to which we consist of our minds or our bodies (e.g., Le Breton, 1988; Plugge, 1970; Turner, 1984), as well as evidence that some people cannot apprehend their body parts as belonging to them (e.g., Litwinski, 1956; Sacks, 1985) are interesting, but the evidence generally suggests that our bodies are central to our identities. Of all the tangible manifestations of self, body and body parts are consistently found to be the most central to identity (Belk, 1987, 1988b; Belk & Austin, 1986; Dixon & Street, 1975; Prelinger, 1959; Vlahos, 1979).

However, not all people see their bodies as equally central to their identities, and not all body parts are seen as equally central to the self. Fulton et al. (1977)

reported that American families were least likely to object to the removal of the spleen, pancreas, liver, and kidneys of their loved ones, and most likely to object to removal of the eyes and heart. Similarly, live donor kidney transplants are relatively common, whereas the less medically risky donation of corneas is virtually nonexistent using live donors. Such findings suggest that certain organs may be more central to the extended self and that they are less likely to be donated because of their centrality.

THE ROLE OF CATHEXIS

Implications for Donation

The centrality of body organs to one's perception of self is related to *cathexis—* the charging of an object, activity, or idea with emotional energy. Women show some tendency to cathect body parts more than do men (Rook, 1985; Secord & Jourard, 1953). Rook (1985) found that more highly cathected body parts are better cared for and that more grooming products involving these body parts are used. Wallendorf and Nelson (1987) provided suggestive evidence that ethnic groups differ in their use of body soothing and body care products depending upon their cathexis of skin, hair, and other parts of the body. Apart from amputation and plastic surgery, our body parts are so definitively a part of us that they are more highly cathected than are material possessions.

This view is consistent with theories that hypothesize that the centrality of various objects to self is dependent on the degree of control we exercise over them (Allport, 1937; McClelland, 1951). Prelinger (1959) also found that feelings of being controlled by certain objects also leads to viewing these objects as more central to our perceptions of self. Whereas it is clear that we exercise a high degree of control over our limbs and the outer parts of our bodies, the very mysteriousness that makes certain body parts sacred may also make them less likely to be seen as central to our identity.

Because visible body parts are central to perceptions of self, losing body parts is like losing one's identity. Those who lose a limb often perceive it as an essential loss of self (Parkes, 1972; Schilder, 1950). Parkes (1975) found that the loss of a limb was remarkably like the loss of a spouse and that amputees remembered their lost limb more frequently than others remembered their deceased spouses. People are also afraid of being less of a person following an amputation. Whereas amputations are generally accidental or surgically necessary to save a person's life, the donation of blood and kidneys, as well as promises to allow other organs to be taken upon death, are voluntary decisions that seem likely to be affected by cathexis. People who rated their general body image as less important to them have been found to be more willing to donate their body organs (Pessemier, Bemmaor, & Hanssens, 1977).

In one study (Belk, 1987, 1988a; Belk & Austin, 1986), people sorted cards representing 96 objects, including body parts, possessions, places, and other people, onto a 4-point scale of "selfness." Body parts, dwelling, and vehicles all scored above the mid-scale self value, and several body parts (skin, genitals, fingers, hands, legs, heart, and eyes) were in the top quartile of scores. Men viewed their livers as more a part of self than did women, while women cathected their eyes, hair, legs, skin, and tears more than did men. Women also rated body-related items such as combs and brushes, dress clothes, jewelry, and perfume as being more central to their identities. Those women who reported a willingness to donate their heart, liver, skin, eyes, and kidney (the latter a live donation to a close relative) had significantly lower cathexis scores for these organs than did those who were not willing to make such donations. For both men and women in the study, those willing to donate these same organs had significantly lower materialism scores than did those who were not willing donors. In this sense the willingness to donate body organs is an act of selflessness beyond the altruism involved; the less a part of the self that organs are seen to be, the more willing the person is to donate these organs to others.

Understanding the role of altruism in organ donation also involves understanding the effect of cathexis of other people and groups as a part of one's extended self. It would be expected, for example, that we should be more willing to donate organs to those other persons seen as more central to our selves. Such donations are tantamount to being gifts to self. In accord with this expectation, those family members with closer relationships to the kidney recipient have been found to be more willing to be tested and to eventually donate a kidney than were more distant relatives (Simmons, Bush, & Klein, 1977). It is also to be expected that those who cathect community more highly would be more willing to donate body organs to others in the community. Support for this interpersonal extended self prediction has been found with blood donation (Titmus, 1970) and with organ donation (Belk & Austin, 1986; Prottas, 1983). Thus, whereas cathexis of body organs appears to create barriers to organ donation, cathexis of specific others and of community appear to create incentives for such donations.

Implications for Transplantation

There is other evidence that transplantation of important body organs can be psychologically traumatic for both donor and recipient. For donors (both live donors and next-of-kin donors for cadavers and brain-dead patients), there may be a fear that part of self is lost in the donation (Simmons, Klein, & Simmons, 1977a). Such fears have been invoked (Barnett, Klassen, McMinimy, & Schwartz, 1987) to explain why appeals to donate organs based on benefits to the self (e.g., "people will think of you as a good and caring person") are more effective in securing willing donors than are more altruistic appeals to help others, as is more commonly assumed to be the major motivation for organ donors (Cleveland, 1975; Fellner & Marshall, 1981; McIntyre et al., 1987).

Transplant recipients have a double fear. First, like the potential donor, they fear a loss of self—in this case because their defective organs are lost. When given the Draw-A-Person Quality Scale, transplant recipients are found to draw smaller and more distorted figures, often with missing body parts (Chaturvedi &

Pant, 1984). Such drawings are interpreted as showing lessened self-esteem, increased insecurity and anxiety, and poor body image. Second, transplant recipients also fear being contaminated by the organs of the other person. When the organs are transplanted from a female sibling, male recipients often fear that they will become homosexual (Basch, 1973; Castelnuovo-Tedesco, 1973). When Blacks receive organs from Whites, there is a similar fear of contamination (Callender, Bayton, Veager, & Clark, 1982). The receipt of organs from another person has also been found to result sometimes in the expectation that the donor's skills (e.g., playing the piano) and traits (e.g., altruism) will also be acquired. The trauma that generally accompanies organ transplantation involves a depression in the recipient that is at least partly due to psychological rather than physiological difficulties in accepting the new organ (Bernstein, 1977; Biorck & Magnusson, 1968; Castelnuovo-Tedesco, 1971; Klein & Simmons, 1977).

CONCLUSION

The preceding discussion suggests that the issues that complicate organ donation and transplantation arise not because of some imbalance in supply and demand, as is suggested by the metaphors of body as machine and body as garden. We instead see our bodies as sacred and as integral to our identities. Only by approaching organ donation and transplantation from these perspectives can we expect to understand the human dimensions involved.

Apart from the moral considerations, it is strategically wise to regard organs as a special category of property that can be given only as a gift. Gift giving is a sacred ritual that is social rather than economic. Cloning, genetic engineering, surrogate motherhood, and harvesting organs or replacing defective parts of the body are all commodity-based terminologies that threaten our perceptions of the body as sacred self. The danger here was anticipated by Titmus:

> Short of examining humankind itself and the institution of slavery—of men and women as market commodities—blood as a living tissue may now constitute in Western societies one of the ultimate tests of where the "social" begins and the "economic" ends. If blood is considered in theory, in law, and is treated in practice as a trading commodity then ultimately human hearts, kidneys, eyes, and other organs of the body may also come to be treated as commodities to be bought and sold in the marketplace. (1970, p. 158)

Another danger that is inherent in the commodity view of organ donation and transplantation is that organs are most likely to be transferred from the poor to the rich (Frank, 1985). This fear seems supported by recent reports of poor Turkish peasants being paid to donate their kidneys in London (Kinsley, 1989). To invoke instead the more appropriate metaphor of organs as parts of the sacred self that cannot be bought and sold at least partly mitigates this concern. Furthermore, appeals to logic (e.g., someone needs the organ and the cadaver is done using it) are likely to be unpersuasive. We must instead recognize the illogical magic and sacred mystery of the human body and perhaps even devise new rituals that preserve and enhance this sacredness. Although we do not yet fully understand the implications of this view for securing organs, it is clear that preserving the sacred life of others, serving a community of which one is an integral part, continuing to control the use of one's body, and achieving a kind of immortality are all appeals that are likely to be more effective than, for instance, pointing out the cost of kidney transplantation (discounted for survival rate) versus the cost of dialysis (e.g., Revkin, 1988).

That the body and its organs are integral to the sacred self also suggests that viewing organ donation as a decision process affected by information processing is another mistaken use of the machine metaphor. In fact, Simmons, Klein, and Simmons (1977b) found that the decision to donate a kidney is really not a decision at all, but a sequential failure of decision-avoidance tactics (e.g., perhaps the tissues will not match). After a series of such decision-avoidance tactics have failed, potential donors feel backed into a corner in which the embarrassment to say *no* has simply become too great. They then *accede* to the donation request rather than *decide* to do so and are influenced by social pressure rather than information concerning the risks and benefits of the donation.

Future research should pursue the metaphors of body as extended self and as sacred more fully. If it is true that individualization is becoming stronger (Belk, 1984; Dickinson, 1987; Macfarlane, 1978) and that sacredness is increasingly attached to the self (Belk et al., 1989; Campbell, 1987), then these metaphors should grow rather than decline in their importance to organ donation. Individual and cross-cultural differences among people regarding the centrality and sacredness of various body organs also need to be better understood. The general phenomenology of organ donation and receipt seems an appropriate starting point for such research. Organ donation could be greatly facilitated if this research discloses that people indeed think of their bodies as machines or gardens rather than as sacred extensions of themselves, but evidence to date strongly points to the opposite conclusion.

References

Allport, G. W. (1937). *Personality: A psychological interpretation.* New York: Holt.

Appadurai, A. (1986). Introduction: Commodities and the politics of value. In A. Appadurai (Ed.), *The social life of things: Commodities in cultural perspective* (pp. 3–63). Cambridge, England: Cambridge University Press.

Barnett, M. A., Klassen, M., McMinimy, V., & Schwartz, L. (1987). The role of self- and other-oriented motivation in the organ donation decision. In M. Wallendorf & P. Anderson (Eds.), *Advances in consumer research* (Vol. 14, pp. 335–337). Provo, UT: Association for Consumer Research.

Basch, S. H. (1973). The intrapsychic integration of a new organ: A clinical study of kidney transplantation. *Psychoanalytic Quarterly, 42,* 364–384.

Belk, R. W. (1984). Cultural and historical differences in concepts of self and their effects on attitudes toward having and giving. In T. Kinnear (Ed.), *Advances in consumer research* (Vol. 11, pp. 753–760). Provo, UT: Association for Consumer Research.

Belk, R. W. (1987). Possessions and the extended sense of self. In J. Umiker-Sebeok (Ed.), *Marketing and semiotics: New directions in the study of signs for sale* (pp. 151–164). Berlin, West Germany: Mouton de Gruyter.

Belk, R. W. (1988a). Possessions and the extended self. *Journal of Consumer Research, 15*(September), 139–168.

Belk, R. W. (1988b). Property, persons, and extended sense of self. In L. Alwitt (Ed.), *Proceedings of the Division of Consumer Psychology,* 95th Annual Convention of the American Psychological Association (pp. 28–33). Eugene, OR: University of Oregon Press.

Belk, R. W., & Austin, M. (1986). Organ donation willingness as a function of extended self and materialism. In M. Venkatesan & W. Lancaster (Eds.), *Advances in health care research* (pp. 84–88) Boston: Health Care Research Association.

Belk, R. W., Wallendorf, M., & Sherry, J. F. Jr., (1989). The sacred and the profane in consumer behavior: Theodicy on the odyssey. *Journal of Consumer Research* (June), pp. 1–38.

Bernstein, D. M. (1977). Psychiatric assessment of the adjustment of transplanted children. In R. G. Simmons, S. Klein, & R. Simmons (Eds.), *Gift of life: The social and psychological impact of organ transplantation* (pp. 119–149). New York: Wiley.

Biorck, G., & Magnusson, G. (1968). The concept of self as experienced by patients with a transplanted kidney. *Acta Medica Scandinavica, 183*, 191–192.

Callender, C. O., Bayton, J. A., Yeager, C., & Clark, J. E. (1982). Attitudes among Blacks toward donating kidneys for transplantation, *Journal of the National Medical Association, 74*(8), 807–809.

Campbell, C. (1987). *The romantic ethic and the spirit of modern consumers.* Oxford: Basil Blackwell.

Castelnuovo-Tedesco, P. (1971). Cardiac surgeons look at transplantation: Interviews with Drs. Cleveland, Cooley, DeBakey, Hallman, and Rochelle. In P. Castelnuovo-Tedesco (Ed.), *Psychiatric aspects of organ transplantation* (pp. 5–16). New York: Grune & Stratton.

Castelnuovo-Tedesco, P. (1973). Organ transplant, body image, psychosis. *Psychoanalytic Quarterly, 42*, 349–363.

Chaturvedi, S. K., & Pant, V. L. (1984). Objective evaluation of body-image of renal transplant recipients, *Journal of Psychological Researches, 28*(1), 4–7.

Cleveland, S. (1975). Personality characteristics, body image and social attitudes of organ transplant donors versus nondonors. *Psychosomatic Medicine, 37*(July/August), 313–319.

Dickinson, R. (1987, April). Self interest: An historical perspective. Paper presented at the Third Conference on Historical Research in Marketing, Michigan State University, East Lansing, MI.

Dixon, S. C., & Street, J. W. (1975). The distinction between self and non-self in children and adolescents. *Journal of Genetic Psychology, 127*, 157–162.

Featherstone, M. (1982). The body in consumer culture. *Theory, Culture, and Society, 1*, 18–33.

Fellner, C. H., & Marshall, J. R. (1981). Kidney donors revisited. In J. P. Rushton & R. M. Sorrentino (Eds.), *Altruism and helping behavior: Social, personality, and developmental perspectives* (pp. 351–366). Hillsdale, NJ: Erlbaum.

Frank, R. H. (1985). *Choosing the right pond: Human behavior and the quest for status* (pp. 192–213). New York: Oxford University Press.

Fulton, J., Fulton, R., & Simmons, R. (1977). The cadaver donor and the gift of life. In R. G. Simmons, S. D. Klein, & R. L. Simmons (Eds.), *Gift of life: The social and psychological impact of organ transplantation* (pp. 338–376). New York: Wiley.

Grange, J. (1985). Place, body and situation. In D. Seamond & R. Mugerauer (Eds.), *Dwelling, place and environment: Towards a phenomenology of person and world* (pp. 71–84). The Hague, the Netherlands: Martinus Nijhoff.

Gregory, C. A. (1980). Gifts to men and gifts to God: Gift exchange and capital accumulation in contemporary Papua. *Man, 15,* 626–652.

Haney, C. A. (1973). Issues and considerations in requesting an anatomical gift. *Social Science and Medicine, 7,* 635–642.

Helman, C. (1988). Dr. Frankenstein and the industrial body. *Anthropology Today, 4*(3), 14–16.

James, W. (1890). *The principles of psychology* (Vol. 1). New York: Holt.

Johnson, M. (1987). *The body in the mind: The bodily basis of meaning imagination, and reason.* Chicago: University of Chicago Press.

Kinsley, M. (1989, March 13). Take my kidney, please. *Time, 133,* p. 88.

Klein, S. D., & Simmons, R. G. (1977). The psychosocial impact of chronic kidney disease of children. In R. G. Simmons, S. D. Klein, & R. L. Simmons (Eds.), *Gift of life: The social and psychological impact of organ transplantation* (pp. 89–118). New York: Wiley.

Kopytoff, I. (1986). The cultural biography of things: Commoditization as process. In A. Appadurai (Ed.), *The social life of things: Commodities in cultural perspective* (pp. 64–91). Cambridge, England: Cambridge University Press.

Laqueur, T. (1983). Bodies, death, and pauper funerals. *Representations, 1*(1), 109–131.

Le Breton, D. (1088). Dualism and renaissance: Sources for a modern representation of the body. *Diogenes, 142*(Summer), 47–69.

Litwinski, L. (1956). Belongingness as a unifying concept in personality investigation, *Acta Psychologica, 12,* 130–135.

Macfarlane, A. (1978). *The origin of English individualism: The family, property and social transitions.* Oxford: Basil Blackwell.

McClelland, D. C. (1951). *Personality.* New York: Holt.

McIntyre, P., Barnett, M. A., Harris, R. J., Shanteau, J., Skowronski, J., & Klassen, M. (1987). Psychological factors influencing decisions to donate organs. In M. Wallendorf & P. Anderson (Eds.), *Advances in consumer research* (Vol. 14, pp. 331–334) Provo, UT: Association for Consumer Research.

Parkes, C. M. (1972). *Bereavement: Studies of grief in adult life.* New York: International Universities Press.

Parkes, C. M. (1975). Psycho-social transitions: Comparison between reactions to loss of a limb and loss of a spouse. *British Journal of Psychiatry, 127* (September), 204–210.

Pessemier, E. A., Bemmaor, A. C., & Hanssens, D. M. (1977). Willingness to supply human body parts: Some empirical results. *Journal of Consumer Research, 47*(January), 131–140.

Plugge, H. (1970). The ambiguity of having and being a body. *Human Inquiries, 10,* 132–139.

Prelinger, E. (1959). Extension and structure of the self, *Journal of Psychology, 47*(January), 13–23.

Prottas, J. M. (1983). Encouraging altruism: Public attitudes and the marketing of organ donation. *Milbank Memorial Fund Quarterly. Health and Society, 61*(2), 278–306.

Ramsey, P. (1970). *The patient as person: Explorations in medical ethics.* New Haven, CT: Yale University Press.

Revkin, A. C. (1988). Organ hunter. *Discover, 9*(2), 64–69.

Rook, D. (1985). Body cathexis and market segmentation. In M. R. Solomon (Ed.), *The psychology of fashion* (pp. 233–242). Lexington, MA: Lexington Press.

Sacks, O. (1985). *The man who mistook his wife for a hat, and other clinical tales.* New York: Harper & Row.

Schilder, P. (1950). *The image and appearance of the human body.* New York: International Universities Press.

Secord, P. F., & S. M. Jourard (1953). The appraisal of body-cathexis: Body cathexis and the self. *Journal of Consulting Psychology, 17*(5), 343–347.

Simmons, R. L., Bush, D., & Klein, S. (1977). The nondonor: Motives and characteristics. In R. G. Simmons, S. D. Klein, & R. L. Simmons (Eds.), *Gift of life: The social and psychological impact of organ transplantation* (pp. 198–232). New York: Wiley.

Simmons, R. L., Klein, S. D., & Simmons, R. L. (1977a). Social and psychological rehabilitation of the adult transplant patient. In R. G. Simmons, S. D. Klein, & R. L. Simmons (Eds.), *Gift of life: The social and psychological impact of organ transplantation* (pp. 48–70). New York: Wiley.

Simmons, R. L., Klein, S. D., & Simmons, R. L. (1977b). Summary and conclusions. In R. G. Simmons, S. D. Klein, & R. L. Simmons (Eds.), *Gift of life: The social and psychological impact of organ transplantation* (pp. 421–457). New York: Wiley.

Thukral, V. K., & Cummins, G. (1987). The vital organ shortage. In R. W. Belk (Ed.), *Advances in nonprofit marketing* (Vol. 2, pp. 159–174). Greenwich, CT: JAI Press.

Titmus, R. M. (1970). *The gift relationship*. London: Allen & Unwin.

Turner, B. S. (1984). *The body and society: Explorations in social theory*. Oxford: Basil Blackwell.

Vlahos, O. (1979). *Body, The ultimate symbol*. New York: Lippincott.

Wallendorf, M., & Nelson, D. (1987). An archaeological examination of ethnic differences in body care rituals. *Psychology and marketing, 3*(January), 273–289.

Wilms, G., Kiefer, S. W., Shanteau, J., & McIntyre, P. (1987). Knowledge of image of body organs: Impact on willingness to donate. In M. Wallendorf & P. Anderson (Eds.), *Advances in consumer research*, (Vol. 14, pp. 338–341). Provo, UT: Association for Consumer Research.

Young, K. (1989). Disembodiment: The phenomenology of the body in medical examinations. *Semiotica, 73*(1/2), 43–66.

CHAPTER 13

ROLE IDENTITY AND ORGAN DONATION:
SOME SUGGESTIONS BASED ON BLOOD DONATION RESEARCH

JANE ALLYN PILIAVIN

There are at least three rather different types of helping behavior involved in organ donation, from the perspective of the person being asked to provide that help: the quite impersonal, essentially cost-free (but also essentially unrewarding) act of signing an organ donor card; the very costly act of being a living donor, almost always of either bone marrow or a kidney; and the highly stressful (although potentially rewarding) decision to allow the use of a loved one's organs. There are many considerations that will be unique to each type of helping. In this chapter I address one factor that is involved in all three, as it is in all human behavior: the self. My contention is that to the extent that potential donors of any of the three categories can be led to see the act as consistent with their self-images (or, in the third case, with their image of how the donor would want to see him- or herself), the likelihood that they will agree to donate will be increased.

I have not done research on organ donation of any of these three types, with the exception of one small study of volunteering to be in a pool for potential bone marrow donors. I have, however, studied blood donation for more than 10 years, and I believe that I have come to understand something about the role of the self in regard to it. In this chapter, then, I discuss the factors that lead to the development of a self-concept that includes the role identity of "regular blood donor," which does indeed lead people to continue as blood donors. My approach was based on both attribution and identity theory; I used attribution theory to help understand the process by which the role identity becomes a part of the self and identity theory to understand how it is maintained and solidified.

A LONGITUDINAL STUDY OF BLOOD DONORS

The data I have used for the main analyses to be presented here come from a longitudinal study of a cohort of blood donors who gave for the first time at the campus blood donation center at the University of Wisconsin from the fall of 1978 to the spring of 1980 (Piliavin & Callero, in press). My colleague and I obtained questionnaires at the time of first donation from 782 of these individuals, measuring their feelings before donation, reasons for donation, initial trigger to donation, reports of the donation experience, feelings after donating, perceptions of the difficulty of giving, and intentions to continue. We obtained intensive interview information, including family background in relationship to blood donation and use, for a smaller sample of these donors. An average of 18 months after their first donation, we contacted the donors by phone, interviewed them briefly, and mailed them a questionnaire. We asked them to tell us about what their intervening donations (if any) had been like and gave them a number of personality and attitude scales. Their total number of blood donations was monitored through December of 1981, using Red Cross records.

Attribution theory suggests that, to the extent that one engages in a behavior under conditions that do not provide an external explanation, one must develop an internal, self-related attribution for the cause of that behavior. A very important variable, then, in our analyses, was the variable that is shown at the upper left of Figure 1, "No external justification at first donation." This was a dichotomous variable: Donors who came in response to a blood drive or who came in at the suggestion of a friend and gave with one other person (whom we assumed was usually that friend) were coded as having external justification for donation, whereas those who came in for other reasons (impulse, seeing or hearing an ad, "always having wanted to," etc.) were coded as having no external justification. Our assumption was that those with no external justification would have to come up with some internal reason for having given.

An analysis not presented here does indicate that, over time, those who continue to give with no external justification are more likely to say that they are giving out of a sense of moral obligation—a clearly internalized motivation. Note that when moral obligation was given as the reason for the first donation, return for a second donation (the dependent variable in the upper right of Figure 1) was more probable. Reporting a family history of donation (also likely to have led to internalization of a desire to give through modeling) and intentions to continue expressed at the first donation were the only other significant predictors of speed of return. Intentions are, of course, generated out of an individual decision process and are therefore related to the self. (Perceiving that one reason for the first donation was "not wanting to disappoint someone who asked"—labeled *social pressure* in Figure 1—is a negative predictor of intentions to donate in the future.)

At the lower right of Figure 1, another dependent variable is depicted: the total number of donations up to the time at which the donor was recontacted by our interviewer. The analysis included only those who gave two or more times.

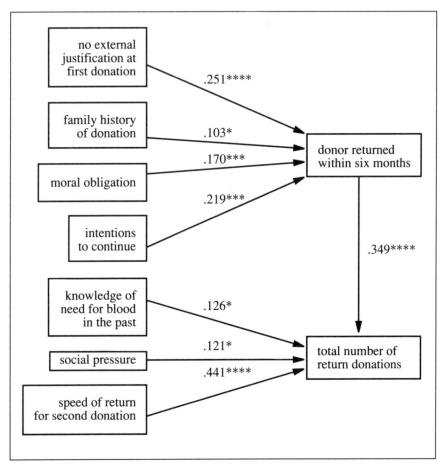

Figure 1 A path analysis showing the probability of a sample of first-time blood donors returning to donate again, based on motivations cited by donors at the first donation. Adapted from Piliavin and Callero (in press) by permission. *$p < .10$. **$p < .05$. ***$p < .01$. ****$p < .001$.

The speed of return for the second donation was clearly the most important factor in the total number of returns, but it was supplemented by a perceived lack of social pressure at the first donation (again an indication of internal motivation) and reporting that someone they had known had needed blood. The main point I would like to make regarding Figure 1 is that most of the effective variables in this path analysis have to do with the self in the sense of the degree of internalized motivation for donation.

Figure 2 shows the probability of return donations among subjects beyond midinterview. Aside from the number of donations already made at the time of the midinterview—a measure of habit—the most important variable predicting continued donation was self-commitment. I conceptualize this variable as involving an internalization of the role of blood donor into the self, such that the person

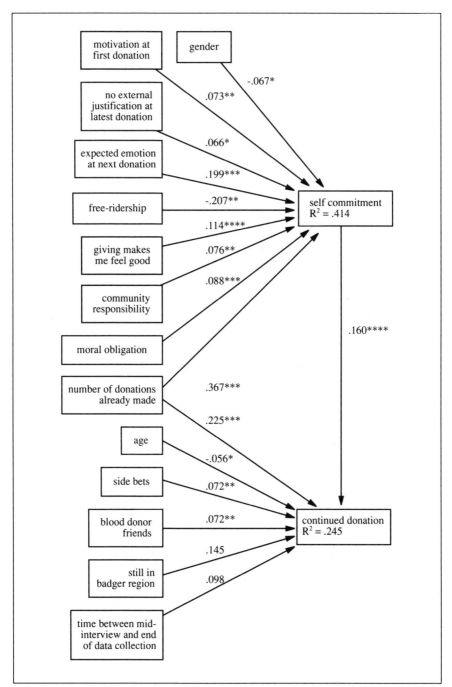

Figure 2 A path analysis showing the likelihood of self-commitment and continued blood donation among a sample of bood donors, based on factors derived through interviews approximately 1 1/2 years after the first donation. Adapted from Piliavin and Callero (in press) by permission. *p < .10. **p < .05. ***p < .01. ****p < .001.

would feel a psychological loss were she or he to stop donating. That is, there would be a little space in the self that was no longer filled with what used to be meaningful activities.[1] A person with high self-commitment should feel that the rule is meaningful and should act out other aspects of the role.

Factors That Predict Self-Commitment

Habit—the number of donations up to the interview at which self-commitment was measured—was the strongest predictor of internalization of the role of blood donor. That is, the more times one performs the act, the more likely one is to think of oneself in terms of the role. Beyond that, however, there are a number of other factors that predicted self-commitment. Two of these were related to emotions: the emotion expected at next donation[2] and reporting that expecting to feel good about donating was a reason for one's most recent donation.[3]

All of the other predictors, with the exception of gender, can be viewed as reflecting attitudes or values. "Free-ridership," the second strongest predictor of self-commitment, is a measure of the extent to which the individual is willing to take responsibility for the provision of a public good—in this case blood—or thinks that it is all right to allow others to contribute without contributing him- or herself. "Community responsibility" and "moral obligation" are measures of the extent to which respondents claim that these were reasons for their most recent donation. In this study, intensity of motivation at the very first donation was a direct predictor of self-commitment, much later on in the donation career. Overall, the first nine predictor variables in Figure 2 predicted 41% of the variation in self-commitment.

Factors That Predict Continued Donorship

None of the factors predicted continuation as a donor beyond the midinterview particularly well (nor up to the midinterview). The two most important factors, however (aside from the structural constraint of whether or not the donor was still

---

1. The scale with which self-commitment was measured leaves something to be desired because it had to be constructed after the data were collected. It is the weighted sum of responses to four questions: strength of motivation to give at the most recent donation, labeling of the self as a regular donor, agreement that one would be disappointed in oneself if one stopped donating, and having participated in recruitment of other donors. Because the last three questions were measured as yes or no, they were weighted twice as heavily as the motivation variable, which was measured on a 7-point Likert scale.

2. This scale measuring the emotion expected at the next donation was made up of the differences between a scale of expected good feelings before donation (e.g., kindly, warmhearted, and energetic) and one of expected bad feelings (e.g., nervous, angry, or skeptical). Donors were simply asked to say to what extent they expected to feel each of those emotions the next time they went to give blood. The scale is highly correlated with the number of prior donations, with donors who have given more times expecting to feel better on arrival at the donation center. However, the scale contributes significantly to the prediction of self-commitment beyond the number of prior donations.

3. The scale measuring feeling good as a reason for donating was made up of responses to two questions asking for reasons for the most recent donation: "I expected giving to make me feel good about myself" and "a feeling of self-satisfaction."

in the region), were the number of donations at the midinterview (habit) and self-commitment. I contend that these two factors are likely to be the most important factors in contributing to any altruistic behavior that can be repeated.

In a later study (Charng, Piliavin, & Callero, 1988), in which my colleagues and I had a much better measure of commitment to the role identity of blood donor, we found that for donors with five or more donations, the only significant predictor of intentions to continue donating was role identity, and the only important predictors of continued donation were intentions, number of blood donor friends, and habit. For those with two to four donations, the only important predictor of intentions was role identity, and intentions was the only variable predicting continued donation. In a very small sample of donors who had given only once, only attitude toward the act of donation—not role identity—predicted intentions, and only perceived social norms predicted continued donation. It is clear, then, that development of the sense of self-in-role can, under some circumstances, take some time. It remains to be seen whether it may be able to be developed vicariously.

Implications for Organ Donation

I believe that the implications of my research on blood donation for increasing the numbers of individuals who are willing to serve as organ donors are different depending upon the kind of organ donation being discussed. Because many types of donation are unlikely to be repeated, prior frequency of engaging in the specific behavior is irrelevant for development of a self-concept as "the kind of person who" would be an organ donor. Nevertheless, I believe that programs aimed at getting individuals involved in other forms of medical helping behavior—such as blood donation—would serve as a basis for generalization to all kinds of organ donation.

Thus, I suggest that any way one can increase the number of blood donors is also likely to increase the number of potential organ donors. It is also possible that simply being exposed to the activity vicariously, through films or television, might serve some of the same purposes. Certainly role-playing has been shown to be effective in related areas. Thus, classes in high school, such as health or driver's education, could be encouraged to provide these vicarious experiences, not only about blood donation but also about organ donation.

A pool of individuals that shows the best potential to be willing to serve either as bone marrow or kidney donors and to sign universal donor cards would seem to be blood donors themselves. In fact, I believe that one is unlikely to be able to elicit the level of commitment necessary to lead individuals to consider living donation by any form of appeal, no matter how self-oriented, unless those individuals come from special populations such as blood donors. Those who have engaged in some other very costly form of helping, such as work with the severely handicapped or inner city youth, may also have developed role identities as committed altruists and could be another potential population. With such groups, I suggest using an appeal stressing the self-image of altruist, the positive emotions they will experience, and possibly the positive reactions of friends. According to one study of volunteers for bone marrow donation (Briggs, Piliavin, Becker, & Lorentzen, 1986), people who are relatively young, unmarried, and male are the most likely to volunteer. Blood bankers are already in the forefront of recruiting potential bone marrow donors, so probably little more needs to be done in that direction with them except to make suggestions regarding appeals they might use to improve their recruitment.

In regard to universal donor cards, I suggest that blood banks be asked to have the cards available at the canteen area at all blood drives and to provide appropriate advertising information. In addition, because committed blood donors are already recruiting others to donate blood and are serving as models to their children through their actions, they could also be very useful as proselytizers for the signing of universal donor cards. These individuals see themselves as in the business of saving lives, and a certain proportion of them might well see recruiting card signers as one more way to pursue that goal.

There are factors other than repeated actions, however, that appear to predict self-commitment: free-ridership attitudes, feelings of community responsibility, and expectations of feeling good about taking the action. Because signing a donor card is an essentially low-cost action, only a minimal level of positive attitudes and motivations toward the act should be required in addition to making the opportunity extremely easy. I suggest including discussions of organ donation in the context of all driver's training courses in high school (and in the private driver's training schools, mandated by law if possible). Aside from presenting the medical facts, including the high need, persuasive communications should be used that stress community responsibility, opposition to free-ridership, and positive feelings associated with the act in an attempt to link it to "feeling good about oneself."

Finally, in approaching the kin of brain-dead potential donors at the time the opportunity occurs, the appeal I suggest, based on the foregoing analysis, is one of altercasting the potential donor as a committed altruist. *Altercasting* is a term from symbolic interaction theory meaning the action of treating a person as if he or she were a certain type of person. Because of the operation of reflected appraisal, doing this presumably leads the individual to behave in such a way as to fulfill the expectations of others that she or he is that sort of person. Doing this in the case of a potential donor who has signed a universal donor card should be easy, because there is evidence from that specific action that the individual was indeed that sort of person. Note that two of the factors found by Perkins (1987) to predict positively one's willingness to donate a loved one's organs were "presence of donor card signed by deceased relative" and "recalled discussion with relative about organ donation." Both the presence of the card and the content of the recalled discussion had already provided evidence to relatives that the brain-dead patient was the kind of person who wanted to engage in this altruistic act.

In the absence of an organ donation card, it will be more difficult to gain the consent to use a loved one's organs, but I suggest that all families should be approached with the assumption that the potential donor was the sort of person who would have wanted to make this contribution had she or he been asked. Convey to the relatives your belief that the potential donor was or would have wanted to be a committed altruist and would want his or her relatives to remember him or her that way. (Barnett, Klassen, McMinimy, & Schwarz, 1987, found that an appeal to "being seen as a good person" was most effective in getting individuals to sign a universal donor card.) In the process, some of the emotional factors and attitudes we have found to be associated with actual commitment (giving makes me feel good, expectations of positive emotions, non-free-ridership, and community responsibility) can be attributed to the potential donor. The agreement to donate the organs can be socially constructed as the final way in which the family can provide their loved one with a positive feeling of having contributed to society.

During the discussions with organ donor procurement personnel that took place at the conference on which this volume is based, it became clear that the most serious problem that procurement personnel face is in the conduct of the interview with the relatives of the potential donor. Specifically, there are often difficulties in getting the relatives to accept the idea that the patient is, indeed, dead. In this connection I offer a suggestion based not on my own work with blood donors but rather on the work of Maynard (in press) on the conveying of bad news. He has studied "informing interviews," in which mental health professionals are providing parents with diagnoses of their children. One of the most consistent and striking findings from this research is that the acceptance of the diagnosis is greatly facilitated if the parents are allowed to provide their own definitions of the situation first. That is, if the parents are encouraged to participate in the process by which the definition is developed, then they are far more likely to accept the eventual, inevitable medical definition. Although this takes more time and considerable skill, it would seem to be the best approach in the donorship situation as well. The relatives should be asked what they think the prognosis for the patient is and then be gently guided to the conclusion that there is no hope of recovery. With that issue settled, the procurement worker can move on to the question of organ donation. A similar procedure of allowing the parents to altercast the patient as an altruist might also be worth trying.

This tactic may sound cynical and manipulative; I certainly do not mean it to. I have read enough newspaper accounts about transplant cases to know that often what the parents will say is, "I'm sure that Joe would have wanted to be able to help someone else. He was that kind of person." They also usually say that it helps them to deal with their grief to know that their child's death has done some good for someone else. To the extent that it really does help the survivors to deal with the loss, persuading them to take the step is an altruistic act in itself. I do not think that an appeal based on the family members' sense of self is appropriate here, because they are not the donors. An appeal that suggests that consenting to harvest the organs will make the relatives feel better would most probably backfire, because it could then be viewed as a selfish act.

As I said at the outset of this chapter, there are a multitude of factors that can contribute to increasing the willingness of individuals to engage in all types of organ donation. Involving aspects of the self-concept is only one; to the extent that it has proven useful in increasing the likelihood of blood donation, it would seem reasonable to at least include it as we are grappling with the problem of organ donation.

References

Barnett, M. A., Klassen, M., McMinimy, V., & Schwarz, L. (1987). The role of self- and other-oriented motivation in the organ donation decision. *Advances in Consumer Research, 14*, 335–337.

Briggs, N. C., Piliavin, J. A., Becker, G. A., & Lorentzen, D. (1986). On willingness to be a bone marrow donor. *Transfusion, 26*(4), 324–330.

Charng, H. W., Piliavin, J. A., & Callero, P. C. (1988). Role identity and reasoned action in the prediciton of repeated behavior. *Social Psychology Quarterly, 51*, 303–317.

Maynard, D. (in press). On co-implicating recipients in the delivery of diagnostic news. In P. Drew & J. Heritage (Eds.), *Talk at work: Interaction in institutional settings.* Cambridge, England: Cambridge University Press.

Perkins, K. A. (1987). The shortage of cadaver donor organs for transplantation: Can psychology help? *American Psychologist, 42*, 921–930.

Piliavin, J. A., & Callero, P. C. (in press). *Giving the gift of life to unnamed strangers: The American community responsibility blood donor.* Baltimore: The Johns Hopkins University Press.

CHAPTER 14

THE USE OF SOCIAL MARKETING TO ENCOURAGE ORGAN DONATION

KAREN F. A. FOX

Demand for donated organs has been created by significant improvements in organ transplantation, the development of cyclosporin to suppress organ rejection, the availability of funding for some organ transplants, and the widely held American values supporting altruism and use of technology. The absence of any one of these elements could significantly reduce or altogether eliminate organ transplantation and thus the demand for organs. With these prerequisites in place, organ transplants are more frequently performed in the United States.

The major constraint now is obtaining an adequate supply of organs. According to Evans (1988), 9,000 kidneys were transplanted in 1986, with 20% of the organs coming from relatives; but 13,000 people need kidney transplants. The gap is far wider for hearts (1,500 recipients in 1986, of 14,500 in need) and livers (1,200 recipients of about 9,000 in need). In the future, advances in tissue preservation will extend the viability of donated organs, and mechanical devices may replace the need for certain human donor organs. But in the short to medium term, donated organs are essential, and the task is to ensure the greatest number of donor organs.

HEALTH-RELATED APPLICATIONS FOR SOCIAL MARKETING

Social marketing appears to be a promising technique to increase the donation of organs for transplantation. Social marketing is the application of marketing tools and concepts to the promotion of beneficial social change—a cause, an idea, or behavior. Social marketing aims to identify and research potential adopters and develop appropriate products and programs that are attractive to potential adopters. These products and programs must be promoted, priced, and distributed in ways that maximize adoption.

In the nearly two decades since the term was introduced, *social marketing* has been applied to a wide variety of societal problems (Fox & Kotler, 1980). The majority of social marketing applications have, however, been in health-related areas. In the United States, successful social marketing programs have addressed reduction of risk factors for heart disease, consistent use of medication to reduce high blood pressure, breast self-examination, seat belt usage, and many others. Social marketing has been widely used in programs sponsored by United States Agency for International Development in Third World countries to enhance the survival of children through promoting birth spacing for improved maternal and child health, oral rehydration therapy to treat diarrheal dehydration, immunization, and improved nutrition through breast-feeding and better weaning foods. Other overseas social marketing programs promote family planning and contraceptive use.

Social marketing found a place in health-related programs because many mass health campaigns have been deemed ineffective (Fox, 1984). Although the mass media broadcast messages about how to be healthier and live longer, health problems seemed to grow faster than the solutions (e.g., more smoking in some population segments, more stress-related behavior, less exercise, etc.). When mass media campaigns did not work, health communicators in the 1960s tended to blame the audience—the public—for being resistant to change, apathetic, busy with other (less important) concerns, even lazy. In the 1970s, some health communicators switched their perspective and sought to understand the reasons why people did *not* act on the "good advice" they received from health professionals. They noted that many people are in fact "rational," that is, "they behave on the basis of the information they have in such a way as to maximize their benefits and minimize their costs" (Udry & Morris, 1971, p. 776).

Social marketing programs in the late 1970s and into the 1980s have been predicated on the idea that people are rational and that they act (modify their behavior or beliefs) because they expect to be better off as a result—that there is a quid pro quo that could be described as an exchange. For example, a smoker may quit in the expectation of enjoying more stamina, a lower risk of heart problems, and a longer life. Exchange by its very nature is voluntary. The two (or more) parties in an exchange expect to benefit as a result of the exchange, and they are free to accept or reject the other party's offer. In contrast, some behavior change efforts have relied on exhortation ("do it, it's good for you") or even coercion. The social marketer eschews exhortation and coercion, instead offering the target audience an exchange that is attractive enough to move them to alter their behavior in the desired direction.

In the United States organ donation is a voluntary, nonmonetary exchange. What is being exchanged? The person who signs a donor care may have a sense of helping others. The donor's family has the opportunity to save a life and thereby symbolically extend the life of the loved one through someone else, which may also assuage the family's grief.

Although social marketing has been used extensively to encourage people to take care of their health and the health of loved ones, it has not yet been enlisted to increase the number of donated organs for transplantation. Admittedly there are distinctions between the two areas of application. Most health-related social marketing programs emphasize the advantages *to the individual* of adopting new health behaviors or of modifying existing ones. In contrast, increasing organ donation depends on influencing the attitudes and behaviors of people who may have no feeling of urgency about taking the desired step (because death—their own or a loved one's—seems remote) or who are in an emotional state in which reasoned decision making can be very difficult (when a loved one is dying). Therefore, social marketing faces special challenges in addressing the task of encouraging organ donation.

TEN STEPS FOR ENCOURAGING ORGAN DONATION

1. Clearly Define the Problem

The social marketer should first ascertain what the problem is and what it is not, who is affected, and in what ways. The end result should be a statement of the issue in behavioral terms. For example, the initial problem statement might be "We don't have enough donated hearts to meet the demand"; the eventual behavioral statement of the problem might be "Neurosurgeons delay or fail to certify brain death, so we are unable to present family members with the option of donation while tissues are still suitable for transplantation." Overly facile or incomplete problem statements can lead to overly simplistic programs. For example, a description that the problem is "Not enough people are donating" might lead to a "Be generous, donate your organs" campaign, which may not address the actual barriers to increasing numbers of donated organs.

The problem statement often grows out of extensive interviews with people who can affect or who are affected by the problem. For example, physicians play a crucial role and are an important audience for social marketing programs. Physicians may choose not to ask relatives for permission to remove transplantable organs because of their concerns about legal and other issues. If the physician does not ask, the relatives do not have an opportunity to decide whether or not to donate.

Problems need to be understood and defined from the point of view of the person who is the target of the social marketing program. For example, campaigns to promote oral rehydration therapy to save the lives of young children with diarrheal dehydration encountered mothers who wanted to "cure" the diarrhea (make it stop) by withholding food and water, traditional healers who believed in using purgatives, and physicians who prescribed useless medicines. The campaign had to teach mothers that dehydration was much more dangerous than the diarrhea itself and to teach traditional healers how to administer oral rehydration therapy instead of harmful purgatives, and to teach physicians that oral rehydration therapy was effective and antibiotics were not (Fox, 1988). Social marketers need insights about how relevant audiences actually perceive the situation and issues in order to plan appropriate interventions.

2. Select the Appropriate Target Audience

The definition of the problem shapes the selection of target audiences. Marketers aim to segment the market, dividing it up into relatively homogeneous subgroups as a basis for developing a marketing program. For example, a program directed to physicians would probably segment the physician market to select those likely to have the greatest impact on the problem. On the assumption that certain categories of physicians will be more likely to be in contact with prospective donors and their families, the social marketer might segment the physician market on the basis of age, medical specialty, board certification, and location of practice (urban, suburban, or rural). Rather than developing one program or one message aimed at all physicians, the social marketer will direct a particular program to a selected group to maximize its impact and effectiveness.

3. Conduct Additional Research on the Target Audience

A number of studies of public attitudes toward organ donation exemplify this kind of research. How do people view the problem? What role do they think they do or could play in changing the situation? What exchange would motivate them and, by extension, people like them to alter their behavior? This information would typically be gathered through individual in-depth interviews or small focused group discussions ("focus groups"). Research that is aimed toward understanding important symbols also plays an important role. For example, Belk (see chapter 12, by R. W. Belk in this volume) explicates the ways in which people think about their bodies and body parts and presents implications for social marketing interventions.

4. Develop a Coordinated, Comprehensive Marketing Plan

Develop a marketing plan that details the four components of the "marketing mix": the product or behavior change to be offered, the "price" involved, where and how the product can be obtained, and the promotional activities to support the marketing plan. Each of these four components is discussed in succeeding steps. The plan should also specify realistic behavioral outcomes, the time frame, and how the outcomes will be assessed. The overall plan is important because coordinated activities directed at a clearly defined target audience are far more likely to be effective than is a single mass campaign directed at everyone.

5. Design and Position the Proposed Behavior Change

Although social marketing programs often aim to influence the acceptability of ideas (such as the value of donating organs), they do not rely on promoting intangible ideas or ideas that are difficult to grasp. Instead, social marketers try to come up with some tangible product that encourages the behavior change or heightens its effectiveness. For example, easy-to-understand pictorial immunization cards encourage illiterate mothers to ensure that their children have received all the necessary vaccinations; providing packets of oral rehydration salts and mixing directions helps mothers and other caregivers respond appropriately to the message "rehydrate your child to prevent death from dehydration" (Fox, 1988).

In the case of organ donation the donor card serves as a reminder of the value of organ donation. Drivers in states where organ donation information appears on the driver's license are reminded each time the driver's license is used for identification.

Positioning involves influencing how people perceive and think about what is being offered. The social marketer aims to encourage exchange by positioning the desired behavior change in a positive way. For example, instead of asking people to consider "donating your corneas when you die," the donation might be described as "giving others the gift of sight." This latter statement does not mislead the prospective donor, but does place the act in a more pleasant and altruistic light, making it easier for most people to think about the need and their own roles as potential donors.

6. Determine and Control the Cost of Adopting the Desired Behavior

In the broadest sense, the price of anything is the cost of obtaining it. The total price includes the time spent shopping, the gasoline and wear-and-tear on the car, the agonizing over which item to buy, the cost of storing and using the item, and disposing of it later. In social marketing the price is often negligible in monetary terms (e.g., signing a donor card), but the nonmonetary price in terms of time, effort, or psychic demands may be very high (Fox, 1980). For example, a donor card may remind the carrier that his or her eventual death is a reality. Or, for the neurosurgeon or other person to ask relatives for permission to remove organs, the cost is overcoming great reluctance to broach the subject of death, let alone asking relatives to give approval for donation.

The exchange principle suggests that people engage in exchange when they expect to be better off as a result, or at least on a par compared to a prior state. We can envision the exchange in terms of a beam resting on a fulcrum, like a seesaw. If the offerings of party A are exactly balanced by the offerings of party B, then an even exchange is possible but will not necessarily take place. Of course an even exchange may be defined differently by each party. If party B's end of the beam is lower than party A's end (B's offer is greater than A's offer), we would say that party A is highly likely to accept the exchange.

This depiction of exchange points out the two ways in which the social marketer can aim to enhance the perceived value of the exchange for a particular individual or target audience. First, the social marketer can aim to increase the perceived value of what is being offered. A hypothetical example would be to assure those who have signed donor cards that they will have a priority for receiving transplanted organs if they need one in the future (see chapter 17, by V. K. Thukral and G. Cummins in this volume). (This alternative to donation based on altruism may prove to have significant drawbacks. It is presented here solely as an illustration.) Second, the social marketer can try to enhance the value of the exchange by reducing the perceived cost. For example, sensitive, practical role-playing experiences may help surgeons to overcome their reluctance to meet with relatives of dead or dying patients and ask their permission for donation.

7. Determine the People and Activities That Need To Interact

The manufacturer of a product needs to arrange a channel of distribution to get the finished product from the plant where it is produced to the customer who will buy and use it. This marketing channel system may involve direct contact between the manufacturer and the customer or, more typically, the intervention of wholesalers and retailers. When a tangible product is involved, the distribution system is sometimes comparable to the distribution system for other products. For example, social marketing programs for contraceptives in developing countries strive to make products conveniently available to their targeted customer groups by providing distribution through multiple outlets (for example, public and private clinics and also pharmacies, open for a substantial number of hours daily) rather than just one outlet that is less convenient. A well-designed distribution system reduces the time-and-effort cost to the consumer.

A well-defined channel system exists to get organs from the point of donation to the recipient. The coordinated system of interaction between a hospital with a prospective donor, the physicians involved, the transplant coordinators, and the receiving hospital constitutes a channel of distribution. The importance of such a channel system is already well recognized and underlies the establishment of the National Organ Procurement and Transplantation Network. Other channel systems are needed to reach physicians, potential donors, and others before this crisis situation. One current example is state motor vehicle departments providing donor cards.

8. Plan a Communications Program

Developing the communications plan is a major task, particularly when mass media communications are often the primary mechanism for achieving the social marketing program's goals. The appropriate audience must be selected, the appropriate messages must be created, and the messages must be embodied in effective communications that are then presented through appropriate media with adequate frequency to reach and influence the intended audience.

Of course, the communications program may include face-to-face instruction or other communications components besides mass media campaigns. In fact, marketing communications include advertising (paid mass media promotion), public relations, and personal contact. Many effective social marketing programs recognize the value of using multiple types of communications to enhance and emphasize the message. For example, the Egyptian national contraceptive social marketing program includes television and radio ads, billboards and bus signs, and rallies (informational meetings on family planning and contraception) held in factories and other workplaces (Fox, 1988).

Many communications opportunities exist to encourage organ donation. For instance, efforts could be made to influence the standard content of obituaries to note organ donation, much as current obituaries request donations to a particular charity in lieu of flowers. The obituary might say that "her eyes were donated to give others the gift of sight" or "her organs were donated so that others might live." Examples of personal contact would be the encounter between the physician or transplant coordinator and the prospective donor's relatives and the work of a volunteer to enlist friends to sign donor cards.

The effects of the communications program need to be tracked, to modify the program (if necessary) and to gauge its impact. A seemingly obvious message can be misconstrued: When former president Ronald Reagan publicized a little girl's urgent need for a liver, 19 people called up to donate their own livers for this child! We can only assume that they did not realize they would have to be dead to donate their livers. Furthermore, we cannot assume that these are the only 19 uninformed people in the United States (see chapter 19, by D. J. Schneider in this volume). If recognized early, an ambiguous message can be modified or replaced.

9. Implement the Social Marketing Program With Professionalism

Implementing the social marketing program will require an adequate number of trained, knowledgeable people who are prepared to direct and monitor program activities. A social marketing program to encourage organ donation must be continuous, because the need for donated organs is continuous. A major one-time campaign may generate increased awareness, but it may not move people to learn how to donate and to take action. Furthermore, awareness fades over time, so reminders are needed.

10. Evaluate the Effectiveness of the Program

Social marketing programs aim to change behavior, but behavior change—in this case, organ donation—is not the only measure of program effectiveness. The social marketer should measure increases in public awareness of the need for donated organs, increases in knowledge of how to donate, and changes in attitudes toward donating one's own organs or those of a relative. The social marketer should also determine which components of the social marketing program were effective, by asking people how they learned about organ donation. A social marketing program that included physicians would monitor statistics on numbers of physicians attending special programs (e.g., on how to request permission to remove organs for transplantation), physicians' attitudes toward donation, and so forth.

The ultimate outcome of a social marketing program to encourage organ donation is an increase in the number of donated organs. Although it is impossible to know how many more families would have donated organs had a request been made, a concerted social marketing program should produce a measurable increase in the number of organs donated. The National Organ Procurement and Transplantation Network keeps statistics on donated organs. If the social marketing program was first carried out in one or a few areas of the country, differences in rates of organ donation should emerge, giving evidence that the social marketing program was having an effect.

THE EFFECTIVENESS OF A SOCIAL MARKETING APPROACH

Groups advocating increased organ donation have conducted campaigns in the past. What reason is there to believe that a social marketing program will be an effective way to increase donation? What particular challenges will a social marketing program face?

Rothschild (1979) investigated general factors that would influence the effectiveness of marketing communications. His hypotheses support the idea that social marketing could be effective in influencing attitudes and behavior regarding organ donation. In general, people can be influenced when they perceive that the personal value to them is greater than the cost, when they are already somewhat inclined toward the value of organ donation, and when they have little or no preexisting resistance to the idea. This set of conditions describes a majority of American adults and suggests areas that a social marketing program would want to emphasize.

Social marketing programs face many challenges (see Bloom & Novelli, 1981). Programs to encourage organ donation are no different. Many people do not perceive organ donation as having any personal value. Some oppose organ donation, whereas others are simply resistant. The social marketing program can do little to influence such people. Programs need to focus on those segments of the population that are most likely to have favorable leanings, striving to move people in these segments toward increased knowledge and willingness to take action by providing evidence that organ donations lead to organ transplants and to the saving of lives. Observing the positive outcomes of a new practice such as organ donation can increase its acceptability (Rogers, 1983).

As biomedical science works to overcome technical limitations to organ transplantation, social scientists—including marketers—should be working to influence the attitudes and behaviors that will increase the availability of organs for transplantation. Social marketing offers promise as a respectful, positive, and effective approach to encourage organ donation.

References

Bloom, P. N., & Novelli, W. D. (1981). Problems and challenges in social marketing. *Journal of Marketing, 45*(2) 79–88.

Evans, R. W. (1988, October). *Donor organ availability: A mirage?* Paper presented at the Conference on Psychological Research on Organ Donation, sponsored by the American Psychological Association; the Public Health Service, U.S. Department of Health and Human Services; and Kansas State University, Manhattan, KS.

Fox, K. F. A. (1980). Time as a component of price in social marketing. In R. Bagozzi, K. Bernhardt, P. Busch, D. Cravens, J. Hair, Jr., & C. Scott (Eds.), *Marketing in the 80's* (pp. 464–467). Chicago: American Marketing Association.

Fox, K. F. A. (1984). The impact of social marketing on mass health promotion campaigns. In S. M. Smith & M. Venkatesan (Eds.), *Advances in health care marketing* (pp. 86–88). Provo, UT: Brigham Young University, Institute of Business Management.

Fox, K. F. A. (1988). Social marketing of oral rehydration therapy and contraceptives in Egypt. *Studies in Family Planning, 19*(2), 95–108.

Fox, K. F. A., & Kotler, P. (1980). The marketing of social causes: The first ten years. *Journal of Marketing, 44*(4), 24–33.

Rogers, E. M. (1983). *Diffusion of innovations* (3rd ed.). New York: Free Press.

Rothschild, M. L. (1979). Marketing communications in non-business situations or why it's so hard to sell brotherhood like soap. *Journal of Marketing, 43*, 11–20.

Udry, R. J., & Morris, N. M. (1971). A spoonful of sugar helps the medicine go down. *American Journal of Public Health, 61*, 776–785.

CHAPTER 15

MEDICAL TECHNOLOGY AND PUBLIC MEANING:
THE CASE OF VIABLE ORGAN TRANSPLANTATION

KEREN AMI JOHNSON

ORGAN TRANSPLANTATION FROM A SOCIOLOGICAL PERSPECTIVE

Americans believe in medical miracles—not in miracles of supernatural healing, but in the rational miracle of scientific, capital-intensive, high-technology procedures. This chapter is about the historical development and public meaning of one such group of miraculous procedures: viable organ transplants.[1] In this chapter, I address the public meaning given to the peculiar requirements of a group of life-extending biomedical technologies. My approach and my conclusions are based on a content analysis conducted (Johnson, 1989) to describe how choices, emphases, and omissions in "objective" mass media reports (Herman & Chomsky, 1988) may shape the demand for a scarce and problematic technology.

I examine these issues from a constructivist perspective, a position that assumes that the public meaning of transplantation, like other forms of knowledge, is socially (as much as scientifically) constructed. From this perspective, I also assume that objective accounts in public media are a source of this social production. Whether professionals and the lay public support, oppose, or are merely indifferent to transplantation, public information about the existence of and requirements for viable organ transplants shapes the meaning of this life-extending technology. Public information itself is influenced by a combination of social patterns that surrounds the development and dissemination of transplantation technology. As these patterns change, they suggest not only an ideological shift in certain courses of medical action related to illness and dying, but also a shift in the everyday meaning of ontological categories like life and death and self and other. Patterns of change associated with transplantation thus include professional debates about the ethics of procuring and allocating organs (Annas, 1984; Caplan, 1987; Daniels, 1985; Fletcher, 1979), practical discussions of reimbursement mechanisms and service management (Davis, 1987; Evans, 1987; Prottas, 1983; Reid & Timmerman, 1987), and how the social reality of once-fanciful themes about a technology advanced enough to conquer death is depicted in literature, radio, television, and popular press (Borgmann, 1984; Pacey, 1983). The following obituary illustrates this last point:

> Elsie Forbes, age 58, of Austin, died Saturday, May 7, 1988. She was a resident of Austin 26 years and a member of Bannockburn Baptist Church. She was employed by Seton Medical Center. Elsie was blessed with a new heart through the grace of God and a gracious person. But due to God's will and other complications she has gone home to Jesus. Rejoice for her! Memorial contributions may be made to Seton Fund-Heart Transplant program. (Staff, 1988).

Even though Elsie Forbes did not survive, advocates of transplantation would be quick to point out that her family continues nonetheless to support these efforts. Given the same information, a social psychologist might invoke theories of attribution or dissonance to explain a request that memorial contributions be made to a heart transplant program controlled by the local hospital. But an intriguing sociological issue is raised by the obituary's suggestion that a group of medical procedures have achieved a separate cultural status: For even a devout Christian family, organ donation and "other complications" are categories now coterminous with—rather than subordinate to—God's will.

Such a categorical shift reflects the social flux and human confusion surrounding the demand for medical innovations in short supply. For the past several years, ethical dilemmas and economic consequences have come to play a bigger part in decisions about technologies like organ transplantation and fetal tissue implants. Although more techniques will depend (like these) on a reliable inventory of high-quality human body parts, many experts dismiss the notion that the nature and requirements of these creations shape society in subtle ways. Yet as information about transplantation is passed from the medical domain to the public sphere, the media unintentionally reflect and modify certain fundamental modes and categories of human relationships. For example, the obituary of Elsie Forbes

---

1. Viable organs are internal organs—like the kidney, liver, heart, pancreas, and lungs—that need a constant supply of blood while they are removed from the body or they will deteriorate. Physicians obtain these organs from individuals who have been declared dead by brain death criteria, but whose heart is kept pumping throughout the surgical excision.

inadvertently expresses a relation between culture (God) and technology (organ transplantation) not manifest in Christian doctrine nor rationally pursued by professionals in medicine, law, or management. In this respect, the obituary illustrates the unanticipated, nonrational outcome of rational plans—the unintended consequences of the development, diffusion, and allocation of a special kind of medical technology.

RESEARCH ON THE ROLE OF SOCIOLOGICAL FACTORS IN TRANSPLANTATION DECISIONS

Taken as the tip of a phenomenological iceberg, the Forbes family's response to their experience with a medical miracle represents a shift in patterns of social activity that is often taken for granted. These patterns reflect invisible social bonds that constitute the shape of society as a whole. The shifts in social structure that I associate with transplantation are manifest not only in vehicles of everyday discourse like Elsie Forbes's obituary but also in professional descriptions of the demographic, attitudinal, or organizational variables associated with transplantation (Kutner, 1987; Perkins, 1987; Prottas, 1985).

In benchmark studies conducted by Simmons, Marine, and Simmons (1977) and Fox and Swayze (1978), these researchers discussed the (often strained) relations of those involved in kidney disease, transplantation, and dialysis. But these studies were not particularly critical of the technology, policies, or role of organizations in the transplantation arena. More recently, Plough (1986) has included such a critique in his detailed discussion of the meaning and impact of the End-Stage Renal Disease Program.

In research pertaining to values inherent in donorship or transplantation, personal (rather than cultural) values tend to be used as a unit of measure (see e.g., Prottas, 1983). With the exception of Belk's studies of the relationship of self to cultural materialism (chapter 12, by R. W. Belk in this volume) and Feldman's discussion of organ donorship as a symbolic cultural phenomenon in Japan (Feldman, 1988), in most studies the individual—represented as an aggregate test score—is the unit of analysis.

Psychologically oriented studies focus on donorship and use more or less sophisticated measures of individual differences in attitudes, intentions, cognition, or behavior (e.g., Barnett, Klassen, McMinimy, & Schwarz, 1987; McIntyre et al., 1987; Pessemier, Bemmaor, & Hanssens, 1978; Wilms, Kiefer, Shanteau, & McIntyre, 1987).

The guiding assumptions of this psychometric research dovetail neatly with the methodology and assumptions of economics (Schwartz, 1986) and offer, as such, a particularly appealing tool for managerial strategies and tactics like segmenting the donor market (Thukral & Cummins, 1986). Although this approach may indeed be useful for planning, difference measures demand an experimental methodology that systematically excludes or imperfectly simulates the confounding impact of an environment of social relationships. For example, the decision to donate organs or to become a candidate for transplantation is not undertaken in isolation. These extraordinarily complex decisions occur in the context of family systems, medical settings, and—most frequently—under disjunct circumstances of extreme stress. All of these factors compromise the generalizability of standard difference measures administered in laboratory settings. To understand transplantation as a social phenomenon, it is therefore important to complement measures of individual difference with a study of common influences upon donors, recipients, and professionals.

A HISTORY OF TRANSPLANTATION AND THE MEDIA

Beginning with the assumption that the media are a source of influence common to all actors in the transplantation arena, I have constructed a detailed chronology of major turning points in the history of transplantation. I based the analysis on accounts in newspapers, popular magazines, and professional journals; on tapes of television shows; and on personal interviews (Johnson, 1989). Using salient events in the chronology as major turning points, I divided the history of transplantation into three general periods.

Period 1: 1950–1967

Viable organ transplantation techniques emerged in popular consciousness with the publicity given to "hero" surgeons who refined life-extending technologies developed during and immediately following World War II. Kidneys were the first viable organ to be successfully transplanted. As national attention was drawn to the specter of heart disease, the promise of cardiovascular surgery (whether for artificial implants or a transplanted human heart) captured the popular imagination and could soon command public resources. Organ rejection was a major problem for both implants and transplants, so the manifest requirement of transplantation surgery appeared to be predictable immunosuppressive medication. Regardless of whether or not suitable pharmacology could be found to prevent rejection of the transplanted organ, two technical requirements of the surgery itself exerted a profound impact upon public perceptions of life and death. These requirements were a mechanical respirator and—except in the case of living, blood-related kidney donors—the availability of one or more high-quality organs from a "neomort" or "heart-beating cadaver."

During transplantation surgery, human organs and mechanical respirators function together to create a novel continuum between life and death in both donor and recipient. Under these circumstances, the presence or absence of human life defies commonsense judgment. Thus transplantation could become an acceptable procedure only when professionals and the lay public had the means to discriminate consistently between the appearance and the reality of death. Once the notion of brain death was introduced, professionals were given the authority to transform death from a natural or religious event into a bureaucratic one. If donor organs were to be available, however, the general public had to perceive this enterprise as legitimate.

During this period, newspapers and magazines included reports of the first artificial respirator, the first kidney transplant, mechanically resuscitated accident or heart attack victims who first were and then were not "dead," unsuccessful xenograft (cross-species transplant) attempts, the first mechanical pump to be installed in a person's chest, the beginning of a federally funded artificial heart program, and the first successful heart transplant.

Period 2: 1968–1980

During this period, the idea of brain death appeared to gain popular and professional credibility, but not without difficulty. Tensions between professionals increased as conflicting rational definitions of life, death, and selfhood were first elaborated, then started to proliferate, and finally became institutionalized (i.e., publicly legitimated). Meanwhile, speculation about transplant-engendered shifts in the existential boundaries between the self and other was confined mainly to the popular press.

Although various definitions of brain death were either adjudicated or established by legislature, many surgeons stopped performing heart and liver transplants. Without suitable pharmacology, rejection of the transplanted organ seemed certain, swift, and fatal (not to mention legally actionable). Because donor kidneys were also in short supply, between 1970 and 1980 there appeared to be a general hiatus in organ transplantation. During this time, however, an unfolding succession of interest group arrangements laid a market-based institutional infrastructure for disseminating transplantation technology. In particular, public funding of the End-Stage Renal Disease Program and the Artificial Heart Program point to changes in the structure of medical practice. These changes reflect the expansion of private corporations from the manufacture of medical equipment and supplies into the delivery of medical services themselves. Although they were not usually a matter of public knowledge, alliances between government and medical industry players led eventually to a means of rendering transplantation technology routine that (even today) reflects the strain between disparate professional perspectives and conflicting political agendas.

Documents from this period included newspaper and magazine reports of the first heart transplant in the United States; the "Harvard Criteria" for defining *brain death*; the first state-legislated rules for transplantation and the declaration of brain death; passage of the Uniform Anatomical Gift Act (which gives individuals the legal right to donate their organs after death); a proliferation of unsuccessful heart transplants around the world; total public financing for the End-Stage Renal Disease Program, which further established an entire artificial organ industry financed by government but controlled by private interests; and the inception of the Independent Organ Procurement Association, a group of not-for-profit, private sector, marketing organizations created for the sole purpose of obtaining and distributing viable organs.

Period 3: 1981–1988

Brain death, an administrative construct, passed from professional into everyday discourse and appeared in novels, short stories, the lyrics of rock songs, and television dramas and satires. Once brain death became a proper focus for black humor or melodrama, the notion seemed to become legitimate in the popular imagination. At the same time, brain-dead individuals were (and still are) an ironic—and frequently unmentioned—source of discomfort and contention among professionals (Youngner et al., 1985). Also, popular notions of self and other continue to reflect inconsistencies between professional and commonsense beliefs about the requirements and effects of life-extending technologies.

Competition among hospitals increased, and viable organ transplantation became a market-niche strategy for service development. Although issues of access and equity were not (and are not yet) resolved, decision makers in health insurance companies responded to a combination of public sentiment and forecasts of potential profit by reimbursing for transplantation. As transplantation thus progressed from being an experimental to a therapeutic technique, the requirements of the technology became bureaucratically legitimated and structurally ensconced.

Newspapers and magazines from this period included: reports of the development of new immunosuppressive medication; the first artificial heart implant; organizational conflicts over the right of physicians to use treatment techniques not yet approved by the Food and Drug Administration; marketing campaigns for organ donorship, which included television spot announcements and bumper stickers with catchy slogans; appeals by the president of the United States and other elected officials on behalf of individual citizens who required viable organs; prepared announcements about a patient's progress that were delivered by spokespersons in charge of public relations at transplant hospitals; the "first" xenograft, tissue from surgically aborted fetuses implanted in geriatric patients with Parkinson's disease; an anencephalic fetus carried to term for the purpose of providing organs for transplants; and the transmission of AIDS via transplanted organs.

CONTENT ANALYSIS OF MEDIA REPORTS

The Coding Apparatus

I performed a content analysis of selected transplantation incidents reported in newspapers and magazines in order to examine the nature of and change in public meaning given to viable organ transplantation over a 21-year period of time (from December 1967, when the first heart transplant was conducted, until 1988). A detailed review of the news reports that I used in constructing the chronology suggested that the presence or absence of four general categories of information constitute the public meaning of transplantation. These categories are (a) information about financial and organizational issues, (b) information about social issues, (c) information about alternatives to viable organ transplant procedures, and (d) information about surgical procedures and outcomes.

Three coders—a female undergraduate, a male graduate student, and a woman who had completed the doctorate—were each trained to use the coding instrument with articles not included in the sample. The training consisted of a 2-hour session that included the vocabulary of and brief history of transplantation, and instruction on how to use the coding instrument. The hypotheses or analytical purpose of the study were not disclosed to the coders. The original coding instrument was pretested and revised until the coefficient of interrater reliability was .90. Three separate coders performed the pretest; these were not the same individuals who coded the articles for analysis, but they were similar in age, gender, and education.

Sample Design

To establish a Period 1 baseline for frequencies in the content categories, one group of 28 articles included all the stories that appeared in the *New York Times* and *Newsweek* about the first heart transplant (December 1967). To examine changes in these categories that occurred during Periods 2 and 3, another group of 28 articles included the complete coverage of local transplants and related events in the *Austin American Statesman* (Austin, Texas) from December 1973 to August 1988. This purposive sample of articles was biased in that the newspaper and magazines selected were all in English, represented a discretionary purchase for consumers, and were not accessible to individuals who could not read.

In addition, those who preferred tabloid news (or no print media at all) were not likely to read these periodicals. Although articles in the sample did not include the whole spectrum of values and beliefs available in the culture, the reputation of each periodical suggested that they represented general and influential ones. The logical flaws inherent in this sort of judgmental selection of specific incidents and periodicals should be partially offset by (a) the comprehensive representation of reports from wire services sent all over the country, (b) the comparatively large circulation of each magazine or newspaper, (c) the inclusion of all articles in each category, and (d) the availability of the data.

Procedure

Each article was coded by all three coders, and I acted as a fourth coder for articles selected at random. The coders' evaluations were combined and tabulated as separate frequencies for each statement on the coding instrument. Sample proportions were calculated for each of four information categories by summing the frequencies of all statements in each category and taking the observed category total as a percentage of the expected category total. The articles about the first heart transplant taken from the *New York Times* and *Newsweek* were then compared to the articles from the *Austin American Statesman* to examine the nature of "objective facts" contained in public reports of transplantation incidents and to see whether the nature of these reports changed over time and, if so, in what categories of information change occurred.

RESULTS OF THE CONTENT ANALYSIS: DOMINANT THEMES

Financial and Organizational Issues

The proportional frequency with which financial and organizational issues were mentioned increased from 1967 to 1973–1988. In the *New York Times* and *Newsweek,* reports of the first transplant and of financial and organizational issues were mentioned a total of 21 times (sample proportion = .04); these were mentioned 44 times in the *Austin American Statesman* (sample proportion = .10). The increase in number of mentions within this general category is attributable to increases in (a) costs to individuals and the federal government, (b) effects of marketing programs or media coverage, and (c) discussion of the activities of transplant coordinators. The frequency with which brain death was mentioned is the same in both subsamples, whereas mentions of abuse of the system decreased from 1967 to 1988.

Social Issues

The frequency with which social issues were mentioned decreased from 1967 to 1973–1988. In reports of the first transplant, social issues were mentioned 116 times in the *New York Times* and *Newsweek* (sample proportion = .12) and 54 times in the *Austin American Statesman* (sample proportion = .08). Although the overall difference between summary measures of the two periods is not large enough to be statistically significant, statements within the category changed both up and down. The number of mentions increased for (a) positive feelings expressed by the donor family, (b) feelings of closeness expressed by the donor family or recipient, and (c) feelings of confusion related to donorship. At the same time, the number of mentions decreased for (a) ethical concerns, (b) racial identification of the donor or recipient, (c) feelings of ambivalence expressed by medical professionals, (d) feelings of challenge expressed by medical professionals, and (e) emotional stress for the recipient family related to continuing care. Mentions of financial stress for the recipient family related to the recipient's continuing care remained the same. Religious issues were mentioned in only 3 of the 72 records of the first transplant, and they were not mentioned at all in any of the records from the *Austin American Statesman.*

Alternatives, Procedures, and Outcomes

Alternatives, mentioned in some form in only 7 of 72 *New York Times* and *Newsweek* records of the first transplant, were not mentioned at all in any records from the *Austin American Statesman.* The frequency with which procedures and outcomes were mentioned decreased from 1967 to 1973–1988. In *New York Times* and *Newsweek* reports of the first transplant, topics related to procedure and outcomes were mentioned a total of 189 times (sample proportion = .26); these were mentioned a total of 57 times in the *Austin American Statesman* (sample proportion = .10). Mentions of differential survival, probability of organ rejection, immunosuppressive medication and its side effects, recipients' daily routines in the hospital, and procedures all decreased. One topic, the fact that a 5-year survival rate is smaller than 1-year survival, increased slightly (it was mentioned in only 3 of 55 records.) In both publications, immunosuppressive medication was mentioned by brand or type twice as frequently as its side effects were mentioned.

DISCUSSION

According to some critics, media sources are not isolated from each other, but refer to each other continuously. Although newspapers, television, radio, film, novels, music, and so forth may all address the same event, the reality of the event is constituted by the interplay of its various representations. With this caveat in mind, the public meaning given to viable organ transplantation in objective news reports depends on the topics that are chosen, how the issues are framed, and the way in which organizational agendas shape the news.

What Topics Are Chosen

Primarily, the topics concern human interest features about individual donors and recipients, the activities of people in large organizations, and—at one time—hero-surgeons. Presently there are almost no features on individual physicians; there is, however, an increasing focus on transplant coordinators or official hospital spokespersons. When transplantation is situated in such complexity, the procedures appear more routine, successful, and predictable than they actually are. Uncertainty regarding the benefits and outcomes of transplantation procedures still exists among professionals in law and ethics, medicine, and public policy. However, the potential for public debate that may exist could be deflected by a failure to mention issues such as alternatives to transplantation, an emergent socioeconomic and racial bias inherent in who donates organs and who receives them, and stress for the recipient and his or her family related to postsurgical care.

How Are Issues Framed?

Until recently, transplantation appeared as a technical spectacle orchestrated by hero-surgeons. The patient's continued survival or abrupt or lingering death was the touch-and-go stuff of public drama. Whatever tension between optimism and uncertainty attends transplantation technology may be indexed, in part, by the frequency with which medical professionals publicly express feelings of challenge or ambivalence. Between 1967 and 1973–1988, the frequency with which feelings of both challenge and ambivalence were mentioned decreased. But in 1967, feelings of challenge were mentioned twice as frequently as feelings of ambivalence. In 1973–1988, feelings of challenge were mentioned four times as frequently as feelings of ambivalence.

By focusing on the wonder of technology and the charisma of those who apparently control it, surgical survival became a familiar public measure of successful outcome. A viable organ transplant does not, however, cure disease. Rather it extends life by trading one chronic disease (of the organ) for another (a chronically compromised immune system). Under these circumstances, the quality of life for those who survive surgery and their families will vary dramatically.

Substantial social and technological problems are still inherent in "the gift of life." Yet, from 1967 to 1973–1988, the proportional mention of differential survival, the probability of organ rejection, and side effects of immunosuppressive medication declined, whereas mentions of financial strain for the recipient's family remained negligible. Omitting issues like these from public reports presents transplantation procedures as less problematic and disruptive than they actually are. For example, the availability of immunosuppressive medicine is mentioned twice as frequently as the potential side effects of these drugs. In some reports, intractable problems of conflicting values and priorities are ignored. In others, they are transformed into issues of uncertain organ supply. An organ shortage is a problem that managers can solve. They develop highly visible marketing programs that (intentionally or not) ignore messy social issues or displace them with themes designed to appeal to individual, private motives.

This tendency suggests that the public perception of transplantation is framed in terms of individual sentiments, not as (still unresolved) broader issues of health and social welfare. Accordingly, costs and ethical concerns were mentioned less frequently in 1973–1988 than they were in 1967, whereas the number of mentions given to positive feelings expressed by the donor family and feelings of closeness expressed by the donor and recipient increased.

How Do Organizational Agendas Shape the News?

Organizations per se are more visible now than they were 20 years ago, principally because of the frequency with which transplant coordinators, marketing directors, and official spokespersons crop up in the news. However, the exact role and interconnections of profit-making firms in the transplantation arena remains obscure. Growth in the scope and sophistication of public relations and news management means a newsworthy corporate image is now de rigueur. However, medical news reporters offer little coherent information about interest group alliances or the market arrangements they forge. The analysis of this sample of articles suggests that complex and problematic social outcomes, debatable public priorities, and details of organizational activities and interests are either omitted or reduced to matters of public sentiment, personal heroics, and an optimistic vision of determinate clinical progress.

References

Annas, G. T. (1984, February). Life, liberty and the pursuit of organ sales. *The Hastings Center Report, 14*, 22–23.

Barnett, M. A., Klassen, M. L., McMinimy, V., & Schwarz, L. (1987). The role of self-
and other-oriented motivation in the organ donation decision. *Advances in Consumer Research*, *14*, 335–337.

Borgmann, A. (1984). *Technology and the character of contemporary Life*. Chicago: The University of Chicago Press.

Caplan, A. (1987). Equity in the selection of recipients for for cardiac transplants, *Circulation*, *75*(1), 10–19.

Daniels, N. (1985). *Just health care*. Cambridge, England: Cambridge University Press.

Davis, F. D. (1987). Coordination of cardiac transplantation: Patient processing and donor organ procurement. *Circulation*, *75*(1), 29–39.

Evans, R. (1987). The economics of heart transplantation. *Circulation*, *75*(1).

Feldman, E. A. (1988). Defining death: Organ transplants, tradition and technology in Japan. *Social Science and Medicine*, *27*(4), 339–343.

Fletcher, J. F. (1979). Wasting human bodies. In *Humanhood: Essays in biomedical ethics* (pp. 65–78). Buffalo, NY: Prometheus Books.

Fox, R. C., & Swayze, J. P. (1978). *The courage to fail: A social view of organ transplants and dialysis*. Chicago: University of Chicago Press.

Herman, E. S., & Chomsky, N. (1988). *Manufacturing consent: The political economy of the mass media*. New York: Pantheon Books.

Johnson, K. A. (1989). *The transplantation complex: An analysis of the relationship between technology, public meaning and social arrangements in viable organ transplantation*. Unpublished doctoral dissertation, University of Texas at Austin.

Kutner, N. G. (1987). Issues in the application of high cost medical technology: The case of organ transplantation. *The Journal of Health and Social Behavior*, *28*, 23–36.

McIntyre, P., Barnett, M. A., Harris, R. J., Shanteau, J., Skowronski, J., & Klassen, M. (1987). Psychological factors influencing decisions to donate organs. *Advances in Consumer Research*, *14*, 331–334.

Pacey, A. (1983). *The culture of technology*. Cambridge: Massachusetts Institute of Technology Press.

Perkins, K. A. (1987). The shortage of cadaver donor organs for transplantation, *American Psychologist*, *42*, 921–930.

Pessemier, E. A., Bemmaor, A. C., & Hanssens, D. M. (1978). Willingness to supply human body parts: Some empirical results. *Journal of Consumer Research*, *4*, 131–140.

Plough, A. L. (1986). *Borrowed time: Artificial organs and the politics of extending lives*. Philadelphia: Temple University Press.

Prottas, J. M. (1983). Encouraging altruism: Public attitudes and the marketing of organ donation. *Milbank Memorial Fund Quarterly. Health and Society*, *61*(2), 278–306.

Prottas, J. M. (1985). Organ procurement in Europe and the United States. *Milbank Memorial Fund Quarterly. Health and Society*, *63*(1).

Reid, B., & Timmerman, E. (1987, Spring). Medico-marketing concerns regarding a commercial system of human organ transplant supply. *Journal of Macromarketing*, *7*, 49–58.

Schwartz, B. (1986). *The battle for human nature*. New York: Norton.

Simmons, R. G., Marine, S. K., & Simmons, R. (1977). *Gift of life: The effect of organ transplantation on individual, family, and societal dynamics*. New York: Wiley.

Staff. (1988, May 8). [obituary]. *Austin American Statesman*, p. C24.

Thukral, V., & Cummins, G. (1986). The vital organ shortage, *Advances in Nonprofit Marketing*, *2*, 159–174.

Wilms, G., Kiefer, S. W., Shanteau, J., & McIntyre, P. (1987). Knowledge and image of body organs: Impact on willingness to donate. *Advances in Consumer Research*, *14*, 338–341.

Youngner, S. J., Allen, M., Bartlett, E. P., Cascorbi, H. F., Hau, T., Jackson, D. L., Mahowald, M. B., & Martin, B.J. (1985). Psychosocial and ethical implications of organ retrieval. *New England Journal of Medicine*, *313*, 321–324.

CHAPTER 16

APPLICABILITY OF HEALTH PROMOTION STRATEGIES TO INCREASING ORGAN DONATION

KENNETH A. PERKINS

Efforts to promote health-maintaining behaviors have increased greatly over the past 20 years, as is shown by the expanding body of literature that exists on health promotion intervention strategies. Although the effectiveness of some of these efforts has sometimes been questionable, particularly relative to their costs (Kaplan, 1984), many health promotion programs have met with significant success. Because similarities exist between behaviors that promote organ donation and behaviors that are traditionally targeted by health-promoting intervention strategies, some aspects of these strategies may be useful in developing specific methods to increase organ donation.

Thus my objectives in this chapter are to (a) evaluate some of the similarities and differences between organ donation and health-promoting behaviors, (b) review some of the types of health promotion strategies that may be applicable for increasing organ donation, and (c) briefly review other considerations that are relevant for implementing these strategies in efforts to increase organ donation.

SIMILARITIES AND DIFFERENCES BETWEEN HEALTH-PROMOTING BEHAVIORS AND ORGAN DONATION

Behaviors traditionally targeted for health promotion intervention strategies include smoking prevention or cessation, dietary modification to decrease intake of calories and saturated fats in order to lower weight and reduce serum cholesterol, increasing exercise, and improving compliance with medication regimens. There are several important similarities between these health-promoting behaviors and organ donation:

❑ The benefits of each will occur at some indefinite point in the future, if at all, rather than immediately.
❑ The temporal "window of opportunity" is fairly long so that even with protracted delays in modifying health behaviors or signing a donor card, some benefit may still be accrued when the behavior is finally changed.
❑ Failure to engage in health behaviors and to agree to donate organs appears to be due, at least in part, to (a) lack of information concerning the impact of each behavior on health or organ availability and (b) lack of knowledge and skills concerning ways to achieve the change in behavior.

There are also many differences between health-promoting behaviors and organ donation, and some of these differences appear to increase ("advantages") whereas other differences decrease ("disadvantages") the chances of success in improving rates of organ donation, relative to the efficacy of health promotion efforts. Two disadvantages of organ donation as a target behavior are as follows:

❑ The direct beneficiary of organ donation is *always* someone else, never the person or family making the donation (although indirect, psychological benefits may be possible).
❑ The time frame for making a decision to donate a relative's organs (as opposed to signing a donor card) is extremely short and has to be made very soon or *not at all*, whereas change in other health-promoting behaviors can provide benefits even if delayed for some time.

Organ donation also appears to have several important advantages over health-promoting behaviors in terms of the potential effectiveness of intervention efforts (Perkins 1987):

❑ Signing a card or agreeing to donate a relative's organs is a single, immediate act, whereas health-promoting behaviors often involve long-standing habits, requiring gradual and comprehensive life-style modification.
❑ There are no side effects to signing a donor card or agreeing to donate a relative's organs, whereas health-promoting behaviors can produce injury or discomfort (e.g., injuries from exercise, nicotine withdrawal after cessation, or expense and time of eating a good diet vs. fast foods).
❑ Organ donation has few if any direct opponents, compared with the established and powerful tobacco, alcohol, and food corporations, which spend billions of dollars to promote unhealthy behaviors.

A REVIEW OF HEALTH PROMOTION INTERVENTION STRATEGIES

Generally, health promotion strategies engage in a two-step approach to increasing health behaviors: (a) educating recipients about the need or benefit for adopting healthy behavior and (b) teaching skills or giving information on steps to take in order to achieve behavior change. These strategies vary widely in terms of target behavior, target population, setting, and scope. Common examples of health promotion programs and strategies that may be useful in increasing organ donation are described in the following sections.

School-Based Programs for Smoking Prevention

A University of Houston program in junior high schools employed videotapes containing peer-aged actors in age-appropriate situations to provide information on smoking and on modeling ways to avoid initiating smoking (Evans, 1985). Messages were focused on the immediate consequences of smoking rather than vague, future health risks. The emphasis of information was toward reinforcing self-attributions of behavior change rather than lecturing or instructing children not to smoke. Results showed a significantly lower rate of smoking in target schools (10%) compared with control schools (18%). School-based interventions may hold particular promise for organ donation efforts because schools are natural agents for education and provide comprehensive coverage of the young population (i.e., nearly everyone attends some high school). Also the young, unfortunately, are potential donors more frequently than are older people.

Work-Site Interventions

Work-site interventions usually involve smoking cessation, weight loss, and exercise. The example to be presented here, however, involves seat belt usage at the General Motors Proving Grounds (Warner & Murt, 1985). In this program, test drivers were first provided brief information on benefits of using seat belts and then asked to sign a card pledging to use belts. A target goal of 60% usage was pre-selected. The card signers were told that, if the goal was met, they would participate in a raffle of prizes. Seat belt usage was monitored on the roads of the facility and compared with previously obtained baseline rates. Results showed that seat belt usage increased from 45% to 70% within 6 weeks. Subsequently, the intervention was repeated, and a goal of 75% was set. Pledge cards were signed by 85% of the drivers, and an 82% usage rate was found over 12 weeks.

Interventions to promote seat belt usage may be more relevant for organ donation than are those for other health behaviors, given the ease of execution of this behavior, although it too requires chronic adherence in order to significantly reduce health risk. More competitive programs have been targeted at weight loss and smoking, in which different, naturally occurring groups within a work site (e.g., cafeteria vs. housekeeping employees in a hospital) or rival companies (e.g., banks in the same location) are pitted against each other, and incentives are provided to the group with the highest rate of successful participation (e.g., Klesges, Vasey, & Glasgow, 1986). One important finding from this research is that group goals may be more powerful in increasing the target behavior of individuals than are individual goals. Such group interventions are also certainly more cost-effective than individual interventions. Work-site programs take advantage of social support, peer influence, and preexisting group loyalties, which may be important because people often find behavior change difficult on their own.

Programs Increasing Compliance With Treatments

Compliance programs may be less relevant for organ donation because benefits are often more obvious and immediate, and interventions are usually intensive and focused on individuals rather than groups. However, as is discussed later, a multistage approach with emphasis on both groups and individuals may be most effective in producing increased organ donation. Compliance has often focused on teens and preteens, such as a program described by Wing and colleagues (Wing, Epstein, Nowalk, & Lamparski, 1986) on children with Type I diabetes. This program involved teaching self-monitoring of glucose, goal setting of frequency of monitoring, and contingency contracting (i.e., concrete rewards for meeting a goal). Results showed substantially improved rates of compliance in monitoring and insulin self-administration, resulting in reduction in risk of severe health consequences. The reinforcement aspect of this program may be effective because, despite the obvious health benefits of compliance in diabetes, children often do not fully comprehend these benefits. Thus, approaches to increasing donor card signing that offer immediate incentives may prove useful for dealing with young groups or those with low donation participation rates (Barach, 1984; Warner & Murt, 1985; Winett, King, & Altman, 1989).

Community-Wide Interventions To Prevent Coronary Heart Disease

Many community-wide primary prevention programs have been described in the literature (e.g., Multiple Risk Factor Intervention Trial [MRFIT], the North Karelia study, the Stanford Five Cities Project, the Framingham study, the Minnesota Heart Health Program). Most of these employ a variety of approaches, particularly work-site, school-based, and mass media. The program to be described here is the Pennsylvania County Health Improvement Program (Stunkard, Felix, & Cohen, 1985). This program involved a county-wide, broad-based array of interventions to modify risk factors for coronary heart disease by increasing blood pressure screening, smoking cessation, exercise, and dietary modification for cholesterol lowering and weight reduction.

The first step involved the use of mass media, primarily to introduce the program to the community, increase knowledge of risk factors, and provide information on specific program activities. Multiple series of messages through radio, local television, newspapers, and billboards were provided to maintain a visible profile. The work-site component included weight loss and smoking cessation competitions among local banks. The school-based intervention involved a brief program of three 45-minute classes on 3 consecutive days. Materials included slides and written information on smoking and weight control, and a follow-up session was included each week for 3 weeks for review and evaluation. Program personnel also contacted health institutions and provided physicians with material to help them be more successful in getting patients to stop smoking, lose weight, and comply with antihypertension medications.

Finally, personnel enlisted the help of volunteer organizations because of their cohesiveness, familiarity with local geography and customs, and low-cost labor. Preliminary results have shown a decrease in the number of people with severe hypertension and an increase in the number of people seeking blood pressure screening. Similar community-wide programs have implemented (a) health fairs, consisting of distribution of information, risk factor screening, and enlistment of participation in formal classes to change risk factors; (b) endorsement of the program by respected community figures; and (c) raffles among participants.

FACTORS TO CONSIDER IN IMPLEMENTING STRATEGIES TO INCREASE ORGAN DONATION

Using a Multistage Approach

As is indicated by the community-wide interventions, single intervention approaches are unlikely to be very successful in isolation. Conversely, presenting a variety of approaches necessarily increases the total cost of the effort. A cost-effective method of combining interventions may be the "hierarchical escalating approach," which has been used to treat obesity (Black & Threlfall, 1986) and decrease speeding by drivers (Van Houten & Nau, 1983). This approach could easily be employed to change other specific target behaviors such as attending health screenings or signing an organ donor card.

In implementing the hierarchical escalating approach, the first step is a broad, low-cost, brief intervention such as use of media, mass mailings, and so forth to present the message to the entire population. Many people may already be predisposed to change and will do so if given the necessary information to act. The shortcoming of this initial step (usually involving media) is the lack of opportunity for recipients of the message to voice concerns and for message providers to respond to those concerns (Alcalay, 1983). Thus, the initial step is necessarily limited to dispensing information and encouraging the already converted.

As is shown in Figure 1, the second and subsequent steps in this approach involve gradually increasing the cost and intensity of interventions, such as more

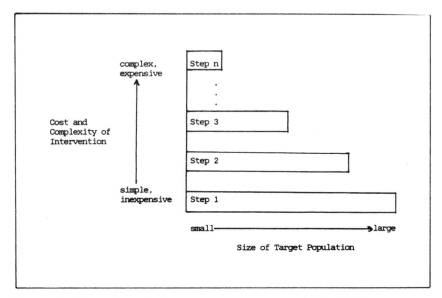

Figure 1 Hierarchical escalating approach to presenting a series of different interventions in the most cost-effective manner. (The content of the initial attempt at intervention [step 1] is simple and inexpensive, and it is presented to as much of the target population as possible. As more and more individuals comply with the desired behavior change, the size of the remaining target population [i.e., those who still have not complied] is reduced. However, subsequent intervention attempts (e.g., step 3, step n) aimed at this shrinking population must be more complex and expensive because the remaining individuals are more resistant to change.)

detailed media presentations, telephone calls, personal mailings, and even face-to-face contact, that are directed toward those who failed to respond to the earlier steps. If most in the population respond favorably early on, the number of individuals targeted by the more costly programs should not be high. In this way, the cost-effectiveness of these efforts will be maximized. This approach is similar to procedures employed in business marketing. Use of a series of short-term, realistic objectives toward a goal has been recommended in the marketing of social causes (Barach, 1984).

In addition to increasing the variety of ways to present the intervention message, methods by which costs of behavior change to participants may be reduced should be emphasized to decrease passive resistance to donation (Weinstein, 1988). Furthermore, as is indicated by the success rates with many of the reward programs (e.g., contingency contracting with diabetic children; Wing et al., 1986), it is important to realize that attitude change may not be necessary in order to obtain behavior change (Barach, 1984).

Differences Among Target Populations
There has recently been a shift in the emphasis of community interventions for smoking cessation and drug prevention toward minority populations because of

the high rates of smoking and drug use in those groups and apparent lack of efficacy of traditional interventions (e.g., Greenberg, Wiggins, & Kutwirt, 1987). Similarly, there is some research showing a large disparity in organ donation rates across particular ethnic or cultural groups (Johnson, et al., 1988; Perez, Matas, & Tellis, 1988). Clearly, low-participation groups should probably receive particular attention, given the substantial need for biologically compatible organs among these groups (Lazda & Blaesing, 1989; Perez et al., 1988) and given the greater room for improvement.

A recent study from Sweden showed that an informative videotape on organ donation had a greater impact in increasing willingness to donate among less educated young men, those with low rates of donor card signing (Gabel, Book, Larsson, & Astrand, 1989). It is important to note that reasons for not participating may differ greatly between low-participation groups, requiring careful preliminary evaluations of obstacles before introducing interventions. In addition, groups may require different approaches tailored to cultural differences. For example, Callender (1987) has suggested that face-to-face efforts and endorsements by community leaders, rather than broader-based, brief media messages, could be particularly effective among Blacks.

Donation Requests to the Next of Kin

As originally conceived, the signed donor card was supposed to be a method of communicating one's wishes regarding organ donation directly to organ procurement personnel in the event of some unforeseen tragedy (Lee & Kissner, 1986). Although the donor card has been clearly ineffective in regard to this purpose (Caplan, 1984), there is some evidence that increasing the rate of donor card signing in the general population may have broad indirect benefits for promoting organ donation.

Specifically, presence of a card for the deceased often sways the next-of-kin's decision in favor of donation, even if he or she personally would not agree to donate his or her own organs (Manninen & Evans, 1985; Prottas, 1983). In addition, individuals are more likely to be family members of a deceased potential donor (and therefore charged with making the decision of whether or not to donate), rather than deceased donors themselves. Signing a card may increase their general commitment to donation and consequently their willingness to donate their relative's organs. Thus, increasing donor card signing remains a worthwhile goal.

Despite the potential indirect benefits of card signing, more attention must be paid to the actual donation request to a family (Perkins, 1987). Making an effective donation request is complicated by the acute emotional crisis in which the family of a deceased potential donor necessarily finds itself. An effective request requires sensitivity and tact on the part of the person making the request (Tolle, Bennett, Hickam, & Benson, 1987). Few untrained medical personnel have the skills necessary for such a task (Koop, 1983). Lack of specific emphasis in teaching organ procurement personnel to make effective donation requests, as

well as an absence of training medical personnel to deal with the general emotional needs of patients and their families, has been a common complaint of
medical educators (e.g. Corlett, 1985; Koop, 1983; Rutter, Mann & Watson,
1989).

Health promotion would appear to have less to offer in overcoming this
critical component of the organ procurement process. However, several researchers in health promotion and psychology are also involved in training medical
personnel to improve their interpersonal effectiveness. For example, some efforts
have been aimed at providing brief psychological training programs to health
professionals in order to increase their understanding of difficulties faced by
terminally ill patients (Razavi, Delvaux, Farvacques, & Robaye, 1988). Other
psychologists have studied effective management of emotional crises and related
problems (Kalafat, 1984).

Regarding organ donation requests, procurement personnel could be trained
to know when to approach the family with the request and to tactfully discuss
with the family the benefits of donation and refute misconceptions (Perkins,
1987). These skills could be made readily available to qualified personnel via
specific training by knowledgable psychologists. At the very least, psychologists
could be useful in providing support to organ procurement personnel themselves,
who often find their job taxing and unrewarding, consequently impairing their
efficacy (Sophie, Salloway, Sorock, Volek, & Merkel, 1983; Tolle et al., 1987).
Providing training to medical personnel for increasing supportiveness and making
effective requests to donate may be the most important contribution by psychology to ameliorating the organ shortage.

In summary, a blueprint for the initial stage of intervention efforts to
increase organ donation may largely exist already in the literature on health
promotion interventions. Careful evaluation of this broad area, as well as of
research aimed at psychological training of medical personnel, will undoubtedly
hasten the development of effective efforts to increase organ donation.

References

Alcalay, R. (1983). The impact of mass communication campaigns in the health field.
    Social Science and Medicine, *17*, 87–94.
Barach, J. A. (1984, July/August). Applying marketing principles to social causes. *Busi-
    ness Horizons*, 65–69.
Black, D. R., & Threlfall, W. E. (1986). A stepped approach to weight control: A minimal
    intervention and a bibliotherapy problem-solving program. *Behavior Therapy*, *17*,
    144–157.
Callender, C. O. (1987). Organ donation in the Black population: Where do we go from
    here? *Transplantation Proceedings*, *19* (Suppl. 2), 36–40.
Caplan, A. L. (1984, October). Organ procurement: It's not in the cards. *The Hastings
    Center Report*, *14*, 9–12.
Corlett, S. (1985). Professional and system barriers to organ donation. *Transplantation
    Proceedings*, *17* (Suppl. 3), 111–122.

Evans, R. I. (1985). Psychologists in health promotion research: General concerns and adolescent smoking prevention. In J. C. Rosen & L. J. Solomon (Eds.), *Prevention in health psychology* (pp. 18–33). Hanover, NH: University Press of New England.

Gabel, H., Book, B., Larsson, M., & Astrand, G. (1989). The attitudes of young men to cadaveric organ donation and transplantation: The influence of background factors and information. *Transplantation Proceedings, 21*, 1413–1414.

Greenberg, M. A., Wiggins, C. L., & Kutwirt, D. M. (1987). Cigarette use among Hispanic and non-Hispanic White school children, Albuquerque, New Mexico. *American Journal of Public Health, 77*, 621–622.

Johnson, L. W., Lum, C. T., Thompson, T., Wilson, J., Urdaneta, M. J. L., & Harris, R. (1988). Mexican-American and Anglo-American attitudes toward organ donation. *Transplantation Proceedings, 20*, 822–825.

Kalafat, J. (1984). Training community psychologists for crisis intervention. *American Journal of Community Psychology, 12*, 241–251.

Kaplan, R. M. (1984). The connection between clinical health promotion and health status. *American Psychologist, 39*, 755–765.

Klesges, R. C., Vasey, M. M., & Glasgow, R. E. (1986). A worksite smoking modification competition: Potential for public health impact. *American Journal of Public Health, 76*, 198–200.

Koop, C. E. (1983). Increasing the supply of solid organs for transplantation. *Public Health Reports, 98*, 566–572.

Lazda, V. A., & Blaesing, M. E. (1989). Is allocation of kidneys on basis of HLA match equitable in multiracial populations? *Transplantation Proceedings, 21*, 1415–1416.

Lee, P. P., & Kissner, P. (1986). Organ donation and the Uniform Anatomical Gift Act. *Surgery, 100*, 867–875.

Manninen, D. L., & Evans, R. W. (1985). Public attitudes and behavior regarding organ donation. *Journal of the American Medical Association, 253*, 3111–3115.

Perez, L. M., Matas, A. J., & Tellis, V. A. (1988). Organ donation in three major U.S. cities by race/ethnicity. *Transplantation Proceedings, 20*, 815.

Perkins, K. A. (1987). The shortage of cadaver donor organs for transplantation: Can psychology help? *American Psychologist, 42*, 921–930.

Prottas, J. M. (1983). Encouraging altruism: Public attitudes and the marketing of organ donation. *Milbank Memorial Fund Quarterly. Health and Society, 61(2)*, 278–306.

Razavi, D., Delvaux, N., Farvacques, C., & Robaye, E. (1988). Immediate effectiveness of brief psychological training for health professionals dealing with terminally ill cancer patients: A controlled study. *Social Science and Medicine, 27*, 369–375.

Rutter, N., Mann, N. P., & Watson, A. R. (1989). Organ donation. *Archives of Disease in Childhood, 64*, 875–878.

Sophie, L. R., Salloway, J. C., Sorock, G., Volek, P., & Merkel, F. K. (1983). Intensive care nurses' perceptions of cadaver organ procurement. *Heart and Lung, 12*, 261–267.

Stunkard, A. J., Felix, F. R. J., & Cohen, R. Y. (1985). Mobilizing a community to promote health: The Pennsylvania County Health Improvement Program (CHIP). In J. C. Rosen & L. J. Solomon (Eds.), *Prevention in health psychology* (pp. 143–190). Hanover, NH: University Press of New England.

Tolle, S. W., Bennett, W. M., Hickam, D. H., & Benson, J. A. (1987). Responsibilities of primary physicians in organ donation. *Annals of Internal Medicine, 106*, 740–744.

Van Houten, R., & Nau, P. A. (1983). Feedback interventions and driving speed: A parametric and comparative analysis. *Journal of Applied Behavior Analysis, 16*, 253–281.

Warner, K. E., & Murt, H. A. (1985). Economic incentives and health behavior. In J. C. Rosen & L. J. Solomon (Eds.), *Prevention in health psychology* (pp. 236–274). Hanover, NH: University Press of New England.

Weinstein, N. D. (1988). The precaution adoption process. *Health Psychology, 7,* 355–386.

Winett, R. A., King, A. C., & Altman, D. (1989). *Health psychology and public health.* New York: Pergamon Press.

Wing, R. R., Epstein, L. H., Nowalk, M. P., & Lamparski, D. M. (1986). Behavioral self-regulation in the treatment of patients with diabetes mellitus. *Psychological Bulletin, 99,* 78–89.

CHAPTER 17

THE VITAL ORGAN SHORTAGE IN THE YEAR 2000:
A NEW PROBLEM AND A NEW PROPOSAL

VINOD K. THUKRAL AND GAYLORD CUMMINS

During the past two decades, shortages of vital organs have been a cause of deep concern in the medical, bioethical, and public policy communities. The many different proposals that have been tried or proposed have focused either on increasing organ availability or on finding ethically and politically more acceptable ways of rationing insufficient supplies. At current levels of need and demand, however, the measures so far proposed are likely to reduce shortages only marginally, and no fully acceptable set of criteria and methods for rationing is likely to be found.

Even as proposals for coping with the current shortages are being debated, the very nature of the problem is changing fundamentally. There is every indication that by the end of this century, the numbers of people who would benefit from transplants will have grown by orders of magnitude, and today's debates will have lost much of their relevance. By that time, we will have been forced to entertain options for increasing supply and rationing that might seem much too radical for today's problems. Our purposes in this chapter are to sketch the changes in character and magnitude of the vital organ shortages that can be expected and to propose a new approach to this new set of problems. We hope in this way to direct study and to debate issues that have so far not been taken seriously enough.

Table 1

CANDIDATES FOR ORGAN TRANSPLANTS, JUNE 17, 1988

Organ Type	Age group				
	0–5	6–10	11–15	16 +	Total
Kidney	74	113	252	12,574	13,013
Heart	13	5	13	849	880
Heart and lung	1	3	2	166	172
Liver	138	26	17	291	472
Lung	1	0	0	26	27
Pancreas	1	0	0	150	151
Totals	228	147	184	14,056	14,715

Note. Data are from United Network for Organ Sharing (American Council on Transplantation, 1988).

ASSESSING FUTURE DEMAND FOR ORGANS

Current shortages of vital organs in the United States are grim by any standards. Approximately 15,000 organ transplants were performed in 1987. As is shown in Table 1, data from the United Network for Organ Sharing indicate that in June 1988, nearly 15,000 patients were on waiting lists (American Council on Transplantation, 1988). Waiting lists include only those patients who qualify financially and also meet the stringent medical criteria used by transplant surgeons. Evans (1988) estimated that in 1987 a total of 60,000 to 100,000 patients who could have benefited from transplants did not receive them.

One of the difficulties in planning strategies for vital organ shortages is the lack of long-term epidemiological studies. We do not know the level of need for vital organs at the turn of the century. The best that we can do is obtain some idea of orders of magnitude through simple extrapolation.

The total number of kidney transplants rose 6.7% per year from 1974 to 1980 and 10.4% from 1980 to 1984. In 1987, there were nearly 100,000 patients who had end-stage renal disease and were on maintenance dialysis. Many of these patients will ultimately qualify for kidney transplants. This population is growing at a rate of 8% to 10% per year. At this rate, there may be more than a quarter of a million people suffering from end-stage renal disease and receiving dialysis treatment at the end of this century. So, if we assume that the growth rate of kidney transplants levels off, which is highly unlikely, at about 13% of dialysis patients per year, the number of people waiting for kidney transplants will jump from the present 13,000 to approximately 32,500 by the year 2000. If

The authors gratefully acknowledge the contribution of Professor Arch Woodside to ideas presented in this chapter.

we take the higher estimates suggested by Evans (1988), the number of patients waiting for kidney transplants may easily reach 60,000 to 100,000. This is a straight trend extrapolation and does not allow for the aging of the population or improvements in technology. These factors are certain to make the shortage much larger than simple extrapolations would indicate.

There has been spectacular growth in heart and liver transplantation over the past few years. These are much newer procedures than kidney transplants. Kidney transplantation became a nonexperimental treatment in the 1960s, and heart transplants followed almost two decades later. Liver transplantation is still considered experimental in many states. In 1987, more than 1,500 heart transplants and 1,200 liver transplants were performed. We cannot make long-term educated projections for transplantation rates of these organs because they are still growing at the phenomenal rates characteristic of very new procedures. However, it is not unreasonable to assume that 100,000 patients could benefit from a heart transplant by the year 2000. The total number of people on waiting lists for transplants at the end of this century could easily be many times what it is today (see Table 1), with the number of potential beneficiaries being several times larger than that.

ALTERNATIVE POLICY APPROACHES FOR COUNTERING ORGAN SHORTAGES

Developing Commercial Markets

The most obvious approach to expanding supply would be to allow private, commercial markets to develop. In 1983, newspapers all over the country were carrying advertisements from people offering to sell their kidneys. One seller wanted to finance a graduate school education. Another saw his "spare" kidney as his only valuable asset and wanted to capitalize by selling it. Dr. H. Barry Jacobs started a "kidney exchange" to put willing sellers in touch with willing buyers. Another entrepreneur, Lance Weddell, opened the Medical Lifeline, which provided cadaver organs for sale to patients in need of transplants. The Medical Lifeline invited potential donors and recipients to register for a fee of $40. A potential buyer had to make an interest-free deposit of $10,000 with the company, to be paid to the donor after the transplant. The company went bankrupt soon after opening its doors, owing to lack of support from the medical community.

In some countries kidneys are still sold on the open market. For example, in one large South Asian country, prior to 1988 one could easily choose one's donor and negotiate the price when the tissue match was successful. But in the United States, the ideological position is that human organs may not be treated as market commodities: They are a special gift, or social commodity, that should not be bought or sold (see chapter 12, by R. W. Belk in this volume). Donors are not to be paid in money, either directly or, for example, through insurance premiums. Through the National Organ Transplant Act of 1984 (Pub. L. No. 98-

507, 98 Stat. 2339 [1984]), Congress closed the door on such ventures. The act prohibits the sale or purchase of any human organ for transplantation in the United States.

Rationing

The supply of human body parts can be matched with demand either by discouraging effective demand or by increasing supply. Because the demand for organs is highly inelastic, it can be significantly restrained only by legislation or by regulation. As an example of the regulatory approach, the state of Massachusetts in 1984 commissioned a task force chaired by George Annas (Edward R. Utley Professor of Health Law, Boston University School of Public Health) to recommend guidelines for regulating heart and liver transplants. The recommendations included stringent criteria for recipient patient selection. Implementation of these criteria would amount to rationing, but they would only slow the growth in organ shortages, not eliminate them in the long run. As transplantation technology improved, and as procedures gained clinical acceptance elsewhere, the criteria would increasingly appear to be arbitrary and inequitable; the regulatory system would be forced to yield to pressure for increasingly less restrictive criteria. Policy would then return to methods to increase organ supplies.

Altruism

Except for the short-lived experiment with commercial markets, we have relied until now on altruistic behavior to expand the supply of vital organs in the United States. In particular, the Uniform Anatomical Gift Act (1968), now in force in all 50 states, rests on the assumption that adequate supply can be ensured by making it easier to give effect to people's dispositions to donate their organs after death (Blumstein, 1989). Previous to the Uniform Anatomical Gift Act, a person could not decide the disposition of his or her own body. One could donate a kidney while still alive, but one had no legal power to donate a kidney from one's own cadaver. Courts did not consider the dead body to be the property of the deceased, and the deceased could therefore not determine its disposition.

It was further held that the next of kin must receive possession of the body immediately after death in the same condition that it was in at the time of death. The order of the right of possession was first the surviving spouse, then the surviving child or children, then the surviving parent or parents, and finally persons in next degree of kinship (Chayet, 1966). These doctrines were serious barriers to donation. The Uniform Anatomical Gift Act overcame them by providing that a signed donor card is to be legally respected after death.

The donor card system by itself, however, has been a failure. Although 80% to 90% of a surveyed population may say that they would be willing to donate their organs, only 10% to 15% actually sign donor cards. In a recent survey, Overcast, Evans, Bowen, Hoe, and Livak (1984) concluded that, although donor cards are a valuable educational tool and greatly ease the problems of transplant coordinators, they are not effective in increasing the total supply of organs for transplantation. Even if a donor has signed a card, hospitals and physicians will not extract organs without the permission of surviving relatives.

Next of kin have from time to time sued hospitals for removing organs in spite of the existence of a valid donor card. Hospitals are not protected from liability if, after removal of the organ, a family member produces an instrument written by the deceased that contains different instructions. Moreover, candidates for organ donation are predominantly young people who have given little thought to dying and have therefore not written a will or signed a donor card. Even if there is a signed donor card, cadaver organs must be salvaged with minimum trauma to the bereaved, which requires their involvement in the decisions that must be made.

The problems with donor cards could in theory be overcome either by increasing the number of signed cards or by increasing the likelihood that a card will be honored. Alternatively, the concept of implied consent addresses the difficulties in persuading large numbers of people to sign donor cards. In effect, donor cards are replaced by nondonor cards: A wish to donate is legally inferred unless the person has explicitly indicated that he or she does *not* wish to donate. Implied consent is in effect in a number of European countries, but with discouraging results. Evidently, physicians continue to feel that they must obtain the consent of surviving family members before proceeding. For the most part, either family members are not approached at all, or they object to organs being donated (Prottas, 1985).

The concept of required request is intended to overcome physicians' reluctance to seek the consent of family members.

> Legislation could be enacted that would require a routine inquiry of available family members as part of the existing procedures in each state for discontinuing life-support measures in hopeless situations. Such a law would mandate that no one on a respirator who might serve as an organ donor could be declared legally dead (assuming that the medical requirements for such a declaration had been met) until a request for donation had been made of any available next of kin or legal proxy. (Caplan, 1984, p. 981)

In the four years since this statement was published, nearly all states have adopted required-request laws. According to the single evaluation that has been done, however, the procurement data for 1987, so far, do not unambiguously support the conclusion that state required-request laws have increased donation.

A NEW PROPOSAL: THE TRANSPLANT CARD

Because what can be realistically expected from policies that rely on altruism falls so far short of what will be needed, we propose that policy be based on self-interest instead. The particular approach that we describe is free of the objections raised against commercial markets but presents new issues of its own. The approach seems to be so attractive in other ways, however, that these issues deserve both research and debate.

We propose specifically that the donor card be repositioned as a "transplant card." Through this card, the signer would enter a transplant network. The card holder would agree to be on both sides of the system: organ receiving and organ supply. With the exception of people already in need, organs would be supplied to cardholders in the order in which they signed up. The proposed scheme has two primary purposes. The first is a dramatic reduction in the organ shortage through increases in supply rather than constraints on demand. The second is to minimize the perceived inequities in the rationing that would be needed under any policy.

The transplant card would be promoted by emphasizing the receiving rather than the giving aspect. In particular, the aim would be to persuade healthy young adults of the benefit from transplantation today, and especially to make them appreciate the growing probability that they would benefit from this technology in the next 15 to 20 years. It would have to be emphasized that they should enter the system now in order to be able to receive an organ from a priority list on a first-come-first-served basis later.

A close analogy to ordinary insurance helps to pinpoint the issues presented by the proposed policy. "Premiums" and "benefits" under the policy would be in kind (organs) rather than in cash. Instead of being paid with certainty today, the premium would be paid only with some probability in the future. For this proposal to work, three principal issues must be addressed: equity, acceptance, and practical implementation.

Ensuring Equity, Acceptance, and Implementation

Equal access to transplant cards would have to be ensured, which means that there would have to be special provision for children and for people with disabilities. Perhaps minors could be included in the parent's card, as is done with passports. Registration of people with disabilities might be coordinated with their registration for the Social Security system.

The financing of the system would involve further issues of equity, which would be identical to those involved in paying for health services generally. At one extreme, there would be no special measures to equalize access to transplant services (as distinct from organs), and the transplant system would contain the same inequities as the larger system. At the other extreme, the program that exists for people with end-stage renal disease could be expanded in both name and coverage to include other organs in addition to kidneys.

Within the priority list for the proposed system, organs would be made available only on the basis of medical need. Difficulties might arise, however, when an organ is not made available to a person with urgent medical need who did not sign up in time. We emphasize that under *any* conceivable policy, there would be people with urgent medical need who would be denied organs. We expect that the number of such instances would be fewer under the proposed policy than under any otherwise acceptable alternative. We believe also that not having signed up in time is as nearly an equitable criterion for denial as any other.

Under existing systems, the most critical transaction for the supply of organs takes place between a transplant coordinator and bereaved family members who have just lost, or are about to lose, a loved one—suddenly, unexpectedly, tragically, and unfairly. The circumstances could hardly be less favorable for an informed, rational decision to help a stranger by consenting to the removal of healthy organs. Under the proposed system, in contrast, there would be no decisions for bereaved family members to make and no ambiguities concerning the intentions of the decedent. In most cases, indeed, the surviving family members would also be cardholders and would thus have made exactly the same commitments as the decedent. Retrieval of the decedent's organs should therefore be much more easily accepted by family members than it is today, and the duties of coordinators and physicians would be merely to inform family members of what was to be done, not to ascertain their wishes or to extract decisions from them.

If the proposed policy were adopted, organ retrieval very likely would become a routine, standard procedure after a person has been declared dead— simply a part of funeral preparations. Just as blood is removed during embalming, usable organs would also be removed. We suggest that the transplant card be implemented as part of a national information network supported and supervised by the federal government. The United Network for Organ Sharing already has a national information network that could be strengthened and used for the purpose.

CONCLUSION

According to any definition, shortages of transplantable vital organs are already acute. Technical advances virtually guarantee that demand will have become many times larger by the end of this century than it is today. Without dramatic increases in supply, no method of rationing will be able to alleviate the ethical or political weight of such huge shortages.

Up to now, efforts to reduce organ shortages by increasing supplies have relied entirely on altruism expressed either through donor cards or through implied consent. Success of these efforts has been hindered by difficulties in getting people to commit themselves explicitly and unequivocally to donation, by reluctance of physicians both to proceed without the consent of family members and to obtain such consent, and by ethical and legal ambiguities in the roles of all of the participants in the ultimate decision to retrieve an organ. Even if all of these difficulties could be overcome, it is doubtful that altruistic motives are strong enough to alleviate more than marginally the shortages that are projected. More intensive effort to tap altruistic motives, such as through required request, will aggravate ethical problems in the system or, through implied consent, will blur distinctions between altruism and coercion.

Because shortages are growing so rapidly, consideration of radical alternatives has become urgent. In this chapter, we have proposed a shift in emphasis from giving to receiving—a new system based on self-interest instead of altruism. Specifically, we have outlined a scheme of government-sponsored, voluntary, in-kind insurance, open on the same terms to everyone. Individuals or families would grant permission to have their organs extracted at death in exchange for a place on a priority list of people eligible to receive organs for transplant. We have argued that under such a system, the legal and ethical ambiguities and dilemmas in existing systems would be eased if not altogether eliminated. Most important, we anticipate that participation rates might very well, and within a short time, be increased from 15% to 20% to 70% to 80%. Thus, a manifold increase in supply could be achieved with no increase in demand.

References

American Council on Transplantation (1988, July–August). Did you know? *Transplant Action,* p. 6. Alexandria, VA: Author.

Blumstein, J. F. (1989). Government's role in organ transplantation policy. *Journal of Health Politics, Policy, and Law. 14*(1), 1–39.

Caplan, A. (1984). Ethical and policy issues in the procurement of cadaver organs for transplantation. *New England Journal of Medicine, 311,* 981–983.

Chayet, N. L. (1966). Consent for autopsy. *New England Journal of Medicine, 274,* 268.

Evans, R. W. (1988, October). *Donor organ availability: A mirage?* Paper presented at the conference on Psychological Research on Organ Donation, sponsored by the American Psychological Association; the Public Health Service, U.S. Department of Health and Human Services; and Kansas State University, Manhattan, KS.

National Organ Transplant Act. Pub. L. No. 98-507, 98 Stat. 2339 (1984).

Overcast, T. D., Evans, R. W., Bowen, L. E., Hoe, M. M., & Livak, C. L. (1984). Problems in the identification of potential organ donors. *Journal of the American Medical Association, 251,* 1559–1562.

Prottas, J. M. (1985). Organ procurement in Europe and the United States. *Milbank Memorial Fund Quarterly. Health and Society, 63,* 94–125.

PART FOUR

RESPONSES

CHAPTER 18

A JUDGMENT/DECISION-MAKING PSYCHOLOGIST RESPONDS

LOLA LOPES

In this response, I would like to comment on some key issues and research directions in the area of organ donation. For the most part, the issues I see as the most interesting are not technical. Instead, I want to focus on the goal of increasing the availability of organs for transplantation. In particular, I will touch on three aspects of the relation between the research in this volume and that goal.

My discussion will be limited to the donation of organs from dead people to strangers and not live donation to relatives. It seems that the circumstances under which a family member chooses to donate a kidney to a loved one who is suffering visibly are so immediate, and so much out of the context of cognition or even moralizing about social values, that the decision is totally unrelated to his or her more general attitudes about organ donation. Therefore, I will discuss only the decision to sign a donor card and the decisions facing the next of kin of deceased donors.

It appears from the research reported in this volume that many people say they are willing to sign donor cards but that sizable numbers of them do not follow through. Perhaps this represents only trivial, logistical reasons such as the failure of the people at the driver's license bureau to point out the signature space to the applicant before the card is laminated. Nevertheless, the discrepancy between attitude and behavior is noteworthy. Many people also say that they would be willing to donate organs of their deceased kinfolk should the need arise, but, in this case too, the actual rate of donations is lower than the attitudinal data suggest.

I think that what J. M. Prottas said at the conference about the highly unusual circumstances of organ donations strongly suggests that researchers who aim at increasing organ donations are going to have to turn their backs on the comfortable world of hypothetical studies and college student subjects and face the necessity, unpleasant though it may be, of studying the decisions of people who have actually lost their loved ones. Researchers should also focus on the decisions of the physicians to support or not to support organ donation. Clearly, this will not be easy. Even physicians who deal frequently with death feel awkward discussing organ donation with next of kin, particularly in the case of the sudden death of a young person. Nevertheless, these are the circumstances in which actual donation decisions are made and in which discrepancies between attitudes and behavior arise.

Next, and still focusing on the practical aspects of organ donation, I would like to note that psychologists for the past 25 years or so—ever since the cognitive revolution started—have focused relentlessly and exclusively on knowledge and cognitive aspects of behavior. Collectively, we tend to see decisions as being driven entirely by what people know. We tend also to think that the only way to change behavior is through changing cognitions. Thus, a cognitive psychologist attempting to increase organ donations would go about it via public education campaigns and the like.

The research discussed in this book (see especially chapter 2 by R. J. Harris et al., in this volume) leads me to favor a different approach. One result in particular seems to have powerful political implications for changing the way that organ donations are made. This is the finding that the most important factor people cite in determining whether or not they believe organs should be donated is whether they believe that the donor would have wanted it that way, either by virtue of existence of a signed donor card or by virtue of inferences drawn from the character of the person while he or she was still living.

As I have become more knowledgeable about the legalities involved in organ donation and in the enforcement of living wills, I have become increasingly amazed that in this land of freedom and independence we don't belong to ourselves. I can give my house to whomever I choose, but not my corneas or my kidneys. I think that if I were to become involved in trying to increase the availability of donor organs, I would use this psychological finding to work politically to change the law that now gives a person no right to say what happens with his or her body after death. The belief in the individual's right of choice in this matter is a powerful piece of psychology because it is something that virtually everyone shares, even those who oppose organ donation for themselves. Surely, political action in this direction is worth pursuing.

My final remark has to do with kinds of research that I think psychologists might do that they are currently not doing. Again, I come back to the fact that most people are not purely cognitive creatures driven only by assessing what they know and adding up the facts. We are also political creatures and social creatures, and there are a great many things that we think about that influence our feelings about social policy. One particularly interesting question having to do with organ donation concerns how a nation chooses to distribute its health dollars and financial resources. I have never seen psychological research directed simply at asking people about their political values.

How shall we spend our health care dollars? I don't know how much lay people know about the costs of organ transplantation, but I believe the costs are very high. More than once when I have seen a tearful mother on television pleading for a liver transplant for an infant, I have had to wonder how the decision to spend many hundreds of thousands of dollars, maybe even millions of dollars, to prolong the life of just that one infant for a few years balances against the decision to cut numerous programs for school lunches or prenatal care for poor mothers as an indirect consequence of that expenditure.

Choices between dramatic individual goods and almost invisible public goods pose difficult questions. Though I sign my organ donor card whenever I renew my driver's license, each time I find myself wondering about such matters. I think that a fertile area for collaboration among psychologists and policy makers is the assessment of people's moral notions about social policy and of the factors influencing their political decision making on these issues. As mentioned previously, I think it may be through political rather than educational efforts that the rate of organ donation will actually increase if, indeed, this is what the public wants.

CHAPTER 19

A SOCIAL PSYCHOLOGIST RESPONDS

DAVID J. SCHNEIDER

Although I have never done research on organ donation, I would like to share my reflections on the chapters in this volume from the standpoint of basic research in social cognition and social psychology.

Generally speaking, approaching the problem of increasing organ donation from the variety of angles represented in this book constitutes the beginning of a fruitful interdisciplinary collaboration. Social cognition, attitude research, personality, sociology, and cross-cultural perspectives all have different, yet nonantagonistic, points to make. Whether these perspectives can be integrated is, of course, another question.

I was also impressed by the variety of research methodologies represented herein. Diversity in this domain is a virtue, but I want to emphasize that several of the chapters, especially those by J. A. Piliavin and by R. Shepherd and H. M. Lefcourt (see chapters 13 and 5, respectively, in this volume) represent methodological directions we could profitably reinforce. I advocate that we think more along the lines of various kinds of structural modeling. Anytime we have a model in which we postulate a series of cognitive and behavioral steps (whether they be knowledge about organ donation, attitudes about the process, decisions to donate, or actual donation), these techniques offer elegant ways to determine what is affecting what. They have historically been used by nonexperimental social scientists, but there is no reason that experimental, manipulated, independent variables cannot also be included in the models.

I would also like to make a couple of points about more general theoretical issues in social cognition. The first is that social cognition researchers, and social psychologists in general, ironically tend to forget about the social context of cognitive activities. When we talk about social cognition we tend to refer to the cognition of social events, and we ignore the other side of cognitive processes, namely social and cultural factors that affect cognition. Many of these chapters have, of course, reminded us that the social context of processing information is crucial.

A second point is that social cognition, and probably cognitive psychology in general, tends to assume that people are rational in their decisions or at least that they take a considered approach to making decisions. It is assumed that people take into account lots of information, plug this information into some equation lying about in the mind for just such occasions, and then reach a pat decision. Yet I strongly suspect that most people don't make most decisions that way most of the time. Many important decisions we make are spur-of-the-moment decisions that require little or no cognitive activity. If one of my children needed me to donate a kidney, I would not have to make any kind of conscious decision—the decision is predetermined by my own values. Other, less momentous decisions seem to be carried by situational pressures. For example, the last time I donated blood, I did so because my wife and I were walking through a shopping mall and came upon a donation booth. She suggested that we both donate, and so I did. I didn't think about it—it was a spontaneous act, albeit prompted by a considerable spousal shove. Cognitive and social psychologists are talking these days a great deal about automatic and controlled cognitive processing. While the kinds of decisions I have been discussing are a long way from true automatic processing, we do need to remind ourselves that many of our decisions are at least semiautomatic in the sense of being quick and requiring little conscious activity.

Finally, let me speak to three substantive questions that have been raised by various papers we have heard. These are: (a) What do people know about organ donation? (b) What are their attitudes about it? (c) What kinds of decisions do they make?

What do people know? Several of the authors in this volume have assured us that almost everyone knows about the need for organ donation. However, we must understand more about what that knowledge is. I am reminded of the story that when President Reagan appeared on television to announce that a certain child needed a liver, several people called to donate their own livers, apparently not comprehending that we each have only a single liver to give up for the Gipper. People may well know that others need organs, but their knowledge about what is involved, how and when such donations are possible, and so forth may be much less precise. Those of us who earn our living teaching ought not to be surprised to learn that knowledge, like attitudes and values, can be skin-deep.

What are people's attitudes? The classic implicit assumption that has existed in attitude research all the way back to Thurstone and beyond is that attitudes are a kind of cognitive possession, something one has, something that stays put more or less permanently. Indeed, most of us probably do have fairly fixed attitudes about George Bush that lie dormant until they are activated at the appropriate times. But I suspect that for most of us, attitudes about donating organs are much less stable. Sometimes one feels a certain way and sometimes another, depending on whom one is with, what one has just heard, and the situation one is in. In the past decade or so, attitude researchers have begun to realize that many attitudes are labile and reflect all sorts of situational pressures. One cannot assume that the attitudes a potential donor has today will be the same as those he or she will have tomorrow, and one is on very dangerous ground indeed when one takes for granted that today's attitudes guide tomorrow's behavior.

Let me propose a couple of research directions based on this analysis, superficial as it has been. First, I would wonder what mental images people have when they are asked their attitudes toward organ donation or when they are asked how willing they would be to sign a donor card. What is the prototypical situation they imagine? Is it helping a young person who has unlimited gifts? Is it helping a housewife and mother live to see her children grow up? Is it helping an overweight alcoholic live to abuse his body further? Modern cognitive psychology has begun to realize that much of our thought deals with prototypical situations, and that, by extension, many of our decisions and attitudes are based on concrete, easily imagined situations. President Reagan, for example, showed a remarkable ability to use concrete stories to persuade—remember the woman on welfare who picked up her checks in a Cadillac—and, whereas many of us may not like the reduction of complex issues to simplistic scenarios, Mr. Reagan's success might encourage our thinking about the role of presenting concrete situations in forming attitudes about organ donation.

Finally, what is the decision? There is now an established body of literature showing that experience with attitude objects, including rehearsing attitudes, not only stabilizes attitudes but also makes them more predictive of attitude-related behavior (Fazio, 1986). One of the implicit issues of this conference is how one can get people who purportedly know about the need for organ donation and have positive attitudes toward it to actually donate. I have been suggesting that most of us have weak and labile attitudes toward donation and that direct experience, including simply reaffirming attitudes, may increase the likelihood that these attitudes will guide behavior. So any form of commitment and of renewals of that commitment, of reminding people and of getting them to remind themselves that they have favorable attitudes toward organ donation, ought to be important.

We should also remember that there are multiple decisions to be made. An important one is getting people to sign donor cards. This is not always easy. One has to get the cards, and, in some states, the signing of the card has to be witnessed. In one of my classes I recently asked how many students carried donor cards—and remember that college students are, in terms of age, health, and knowledge a primary pool of donors—and only 2 of 50 students did. Many of them reported that they had intended to get the cards, and others reported that they had the cards but had never remembered to get them signed; a couple were signed but not witnessed. Obviously there are a series of relatively inconsequential steps here, and relatively trivial inconveniences at each may remove people from the pool.

Finally, we must remember that such decisions are corporate, in the sense that, after a potential donor's death, the family generally must agree to honor the donor's request. Kurt Lewin's classic but often-forgotten research alerted social psychologists to the importance of having groups make decisions that affect all concerned. Families ought to discuss these issues as a part of a larger set of issues about death and dying. There are a variety of contexts in which this could happen outside the home—church and service groups come to mind. When the family of a potential donor is clear about the donor's wishes, there is no need to negotiate a decision at the point at which a physician or transplant coordinator approaches the family after the death of the donor. I realize that setting up discussion groups for the purposes of getting organ donation decisions is impractical on a large enough scale to make a real difference. But my point is a more general one. Organ donation is part of a much larger set of issues surrounding death, and I would like to think that our society is moving toward greater recognition that such issues must be discussed openly. When that happens, the organ donation question may take care of itself.

Reference

Fazio, R. H. (1986). How do attitudes guide behavior? In R. M. Sorrentino & E. T. Higgins (Eds.), *Handbook of motivation and cognition*. New York: Guilford Press.

CHAPTER 20

A POLICY RESEARCH
PSYCHOLOGIST RESPONDS

KENNETH R. HAMMOND

As I understand the purpose of the conference and the book, it is to explore the potential contribution of psychological research to problems associated with organ transplantation. Without any reservation at all, I can see that some psychological research will provide a good deal of intellectual interest, will help us to understand what people have referred to as underlying relationships, and will provide everyone with a more differentiated view of the problem of increasing donation. Somewhat more specifically, it will probably help kill a number of myths and thus clarify our conception of the problem. However, I don't see how it will help reduce the shortfall of donor organs, about which I will comment later. Now I want to make some specific suggestions for administrators and psychologists.

To administrators, I say: Stop doing variable-based research. That is, stop gathering data that tells us that such-and-such percent of such-and-such a class does this, that, or the other. That type of information is practically useless for people who have to engage in policy-making. By the time the policymaker gets down to the bottom of the tree with all of those little branches, the policymaker can only put that information together in an intuitive fashion; overwhelmed by all the little boxes with all those numbers, the policymaker usually bases his or her decision on one or two of the branches, or on none at all (e.g., Brunner, Fitch, Grassia, Kathleen, & Hammond, 1987).

What should be done instead? Administrators should demand that researchers make use of cluster analysis, which provides an identification of various *groups* of people who have characteristics that hold them together: I did a mental cluster analysis of the demographic information about typical organ donors and recipients, and I came up with the conclusion that the donor group consists of poor, Black, uneducated, young males, whereas the recipient group is middle-class, White, with a wide age distribution, and educated. Obviously that kind of give-and-take relationship—if it's real—raises some political and policy issues that have to be addressed. My suggestion for the administrators, then, is that they stop using variable-based analysis of populations and use cluster analysis instead, so that they can find out if that relationship is real.

I suggest to the psychologists that they recognize that there is a difference between "cold judgments" and "hot judgments." Hot judgments are made when people are in difficult emotional circumstances, and their judgments are likely to be made very rapidly. If it is true that the critical decision about donation is made by the next of kin at the deathbed—some of the chapters indicate this, but others tend to ignore the matter—then psychologists must face up to the fact that administrators and policymakers aren't going to pay much attention to their research if it is done with college students in relatively cool, that is, benign, circumstances. That problem won't be easy to solve, but there is no point in working on the wrong problem.

Where, then, is the bottleneck? With respect to the shortfall of organs, the administrators that I talked to at the conference indicate that the problem really is not with the public but with the doctors. But few of the chapters in this volume address the question of the doctor's judgment in this problem. That seems odd, because the administrators at the conference told me that that is where the real problem is. Even if the donations or willingness to donate on the part of the public increased a great deal, they say, very little would change with respect to the supply of organs. That is because the doctors constitute a bottleneck. I was also told that they already know why the doctors are a bottleneck and that there really isn't much being done to address that issue. That is exactly the kind of problem that can be researched and one that is apt to turn up useful information. The claim that doctors are the bottleneck may turn out to be a myth, but, if so, then that is a myth that needs to be killed by research. One often gets surprises when researching such issues.

Let me conclude with the observation that the academics and the administrators should work on a more frank and realistic basis than they have so far. I think it is possible to go beyond academic exercises, but the academics are going to have to demonstrate how their research will enable us to do that.

Reference

Brunner, R., Fitch, S., Grassia, J., Kathleen, L., & Hammond, K. (1987). Improving data utilization: The case-wise alternative. *Policy Sciences*, *20*, 365–394.

CHAPTER 21

CONCLUSION:
WE'VE ONLY JUST BEGUN

RICHARD JACKSON HARRIS AND JAMES SHANTEAU

As we mentioned in the introduction, this is the first volume of writings by scholars studying organ donation from a psychological perspective. As might be expected in such a new endeavor, knowledge is accumulating very quickly, and basic assumptions and methods are being frequently questioned and revised. We thus run the risk of the research reported here being obsolete before it is even published. Even now, we have this gnawing feeling that, in a few years, the work reported in this volume may be seen as quaintly naive and seriously flawed.

Still, this book offers an important beginning. If these chapters can serve as the catalyst to foster more definitive research and thinking that can have a salutary impact on the scarcity of donor organs, then that purpose alone will be a substantial one. In this final chapter, we will briefly describe some possibly fruitful directions for future research. These ideas are not entirely our own and in most cases were suggested by participants at the conference.

On the morning of the second day of the conference, the transplant specialists and coordinators participated in a panel discussion to respond to the papers presented the previous day and contained in this volume. Under the leadership of Edi Servino of the United Network of Organ Sharing (UNOS), a framework for future research was sketched out. There seemed to be consensus of those at the conference that, although laboratory research can be very helpful, especially in early stages of studying this problem, we will have to increasingly examine donation decisions in the real world (see chapter 18 by L. Lopes and chapter 19 by D. J. Schneider, in this volume, for arguments on this point).

RESEARCH DEVELOPMENTS

Three subject populations were identified for future study. First are donor families, particularly those who had already participated in such a decision. (Sometimes, however, it might also be appropriate to study potential donor families, especially insofar as it is reasonable to compare their responses with those of actual donor families.) A second subject group are the health professionals, especially neurosurgeons, intensive care unit (ICU) and emergency room nurses, and possibly hospital administrators. Finally, a third group consists of nonmedical professionals who may be facilitators of the donation decision, primarily transplant coordinators but perhaps also hospital chaplains and other clergy.

Each of these subject groups may be studied in what can be termed the "pre-event," "intraevent," or "postevent" time frame, depending on the temporal context of the donation decision by the next of kin. For example, pre-event problems could deal with public education for potential donor families, as well as more sharply focused professional education efforts for medical and transplant professionals. More effectively encouraging people to sign donor cards as an unequivocal public statement of intent would be part of such an approach.

Intraevent research would focus on the actual decision making in the hospital crisis situation. This would include issues such as family group dynamics, how the medical professional should approach the donor family, what sort of language is most helpful in explaining brain death and requesting organ donation, and how the personal inadequacies and situational discomfort of the professionals enter into their behavior. Helping the professionals to better understand the psychology of people's crisis functioning and decision making would also be helpful.

Postevent research would consist of follow-up work on donor families to discover what kind of information they have found helpful, how the donation decision (for or against) has affected subsequent coping with grief, and how public they feel information about donors and recipients should be. Postevent research on health and other professionals would examine their continuing adjustment to the tasks they must perform, how to avoid burnout and cynicism, and how generally to affirm their own roles in the transplant process.

One trend likely to grow is the increasing use of more specialized subject populations. Early work from a cognitive or marketing perspective can make worthwhile use of data from the general public (often translated in the real world of academic research to be college students). We expect to see more study of donor families and the various groups of health professionals involved with the organ procurement and transplantation processes. As an example of such research, Prottas and Batten (1988) assessed the knowledge and attitudes of neurosurgeons, hospital administrators, ICU nurses, and directors of nursing. Youngner, Landefeld, Coulton, Juknialis, and Leary (1989) assessed medical professionals' knowledge of brain death.

CONCEPTUAL DEVELOPMENTS

In terms of theoretical orientation, the psychological research on organ donation is presently largely atheoretical, a state not unusual for new applied research areas. Still, various theoretical approaches have made their contributions to particular projects in this volume, including information integration (see chapter 6 by J. Shanteau and J. J. Skowronski), social cognition (see chapter 5 by R. Shepherd and H. M. Lefcourt), and path analysis (see chapter 13 by J. A. Piliavin and chapter 3 by B. E. Nolan and P. J. McGrath). As the field matures, one may expect better definition from specific theoretical frameworks, with the possible emergence of a unique theoretical view or a more enduring eclectic situation.

A perspective largely absent in the literature (except see chapter 7 by D. J. Hessing, in this volume), but likely to become more important, is a cross-national and cross-cultural perspective on issues of organ donation and transplantation. These issues are being handled in many different societies of the world in diverse ways, not always with full benefit of the knowledge and mistakes experienced elsewhere (e.g., Daar, 1989; Feldman, 1988; Martinez & Pereyra, 1987; Veatch, 1989; Wight, 1988). Progress in some nations is hampered by lack of an accepted or legal definition of *brain death* (e.g., Toshiro, 1989; Ohi et al., 1986). Certain legislation and medical practices are acceptable in one society but not in another for reasons of culture, law, or tradition. For example, different religious teachings and perceived religious views, even if misapplied, are part of the reality of the social acceptance of organ donation (Cohen, 1988; May, 1988; Moran, 1986; Sachedina, 1988; Tsuji, 1988; Ulshafer, 1988; Walters, 1988; Weiss, 1988).

Though not the topic of this volume, the parallel legal and legislative issues are constantly changing and necessarily interact with the psychological questions of interest. For example, the legislation of a required request policy changes the focus from how to encourage people to sign donor cards to how to ask them to request consent from next of kin for the donation (Andersen & Fox, 1988; Caplan, 1984; Conley, 1988; Martyn, Wright, & Clark, 1988; Novick & Epstein, 1987). Possible legislation concerning the use of fetal tissue in brain implants will help to shape the most important psychological questions regarding the technology of brain tissue transplants. The hotly debated current controversy over the use of anencephalic infants as donors looms as a major issue in organ transplantation over the next few years. (See Annas & Elias, 1989; Caplan, 1988; Capron, 1987; Davis, 1988; Fletcher, Robertson, & Harrison, 1986; Greely et al., 1989; Harrison & Meilaender, 1986; Leggans, 1988; Shewmon, Capron, Peacock, & Schulman, 1989; Walters and Asheval, 1989; Willis, 1988; and Zaner, 1989 for discussions of this issue.)

In closing, then, we consider this book of readings to be a landmark collection of work on psychological research on organ donation. It is a landmark, however, simply because it is the first. We see its value primarily as a stimulus to further thought and research on the topic. Many of the chapters herein contain what is essentially pilot research and initial formalization of thinking. We have great hope that work to follow, in the long and even in the short term, will be far more sophisticated in methodology, definitive in conclusions, and far-reaching in social ramifications. Still, such work will need the chapters in this volume as a base.

References

Andersen, K. S., & Fox, D. M. (1988). The impact of routine inquiry laws on organ donations. *Health Affairs, 7*(5), 65–78.

Annas, G. J., & Elias, S. (1989). The politics of transplantation of human fetal tissue. *New England Journal of Medicine, 320*(16), 1079–1082.

Caplan, A. L. (1984, October). Organ procurement: It's not in the cards. *The Hastings Center Report, 14*, 9–12.

Caplan, A. L. (1988). Ethical issues in the use of anencephalic infants as a source of organs and tissues for transplantation. *Transplantation Proceedings, 20*(4, Suppl. 5), 42–49.

Capron, A. M. (1987, February). Anencephalic donors: Separate the dead from the dying. *The Hastings Center Report, 17*, 5–9.

Cohen, K. S. (1988). Choose life: Jewish tradition and organ transplantation. *Delaware Medical Journal, 60*(9), 509–511.

Conley, D. (1988, June). DHHS-funded study of required request's impact on organ procurement reported. *Nephrology News and Issues*, pp. 32–41.

Daar, A. S. (1989). Ethical issues: A Middle East perspective. *Transplantation Proceedings, 21*(1), 1402–1404.

Davis, A. (1988). The status of anencephalic babies: Should their bodies be used as donor banks? *Journal of Medical Ethics, 14*, 150–153.

Feldman, E. A. (1988). Defining death: Organ transplants, tradition and technology in Japan. *Social Science and Medicine, 27*(4), 339–343.

Fletcher, J. C., Robertson, J. A., & Harrison, M. R. (1986). Primates and anencephalics as sources for pediatric organ transplants: Medical, legal, and ethical issues. *Fetal Therapy, 1*(2–3), 150–164.

Greely, H. T., Hamm, T., Johnson, R., Price, C. R., Weingarten, R., & Raffin, T. (1989). The ethical use of human fetal tissue in medicine. *New England Journal of Medicine, 320*(16), 1093–1096.

Harrison, M. R., & Meilaender, G. (1986, April). The anencephalic newborn as organ donor: Legal and ethical perspectives. *The Hastings Center Report, 16*, 21–23.

Leggans, T. (1988). Anencephalic infants as organ donors: Legal and ethical perspectives. *Journal of Legal Medicine, 9*(3), 449–465.

Martinez, L., & Pereyra, J. (1987). Renal transplantation in South America. *Transplantation Proceedings, 19*, 3642–3644.

Martyn, S., Wright, R., & Clark, L. (1986). Required request for organ donation: Moral, clinical, and legal problems. *The Hastings Center Report, 18*, 27–34.

May, W. F. (1988). Religious obstacles and warrants for the donation of body parts. *Transplantation Proceedings, 20*(1, Suppl. 1), 1079–1083.

Moran, M. (1986). Acting out faith through organ donation, *The Christian Century, 103*, 572–573.

Novick, A. C., & Epstein, F. (1987). The need for mandatory organ donor request. *Cleveland Clinic Journal of Medicine, 54*(3), 163–164.

Ohi, G., Hasegawa, T., Kumano, H., Kai, I., Takenaga, N., Taguchi, Y., Saito, H., & Ino, T. (1986). Why are cadaveric renal transplants so hard to find in Japan? An analysis of economic and attitudinal aspects. *Health Policy, 6*(3), 269–278.

Prottas, J., & Batten, H. L. (1988). Health professionals and hospital administrators in organ procurement: Attitudes, reservations, and their resolutions. *American Journal of Public Health, 78*, 642–645.

Sachedina, A. A. (1988). Islamic views on organ transplantation. *Transplantation Proceedings, 20*(1, Suppl. 1), 1084–1088.

Shewmon, D. A., Capron, A. M., Peacock, W. S., & Schulman, B. L. (1989). The use of anencephalic infants as organ sources: A critique. *Journal of the American Medical Association, 261*(12), 1773–1781.

Toshiro, U. (1989). Transplants forbidden. *Japan Quarterly, 36*(2), 146–154.

Tsuji, K. T. (1988). The Buddhist view of the body and organ transplantation. *Transplantation Proceedings, 20*(1, Suppl. 1), 1076–1078.

Ulshafer, T. R. (1988). A Catholic perspective on religion and organ transplantation. *Delaware Medical Journal 60*(9), 505–507.

Veatch, R. M. (1989). Medical ethics in the Soviet Union. *The Hastings Center Report, 19*(2), 11–14.

Walters, J. W., & Asheval, S. (1989). Anencephalic infants as organ donors and the brain death standard. *Journal of Medicine and Philosophy, 14*(1), 79–87.

Walters, M. (1988). John 15:13: A Protestant's views of organ donation. *Delaware Medical Journal, 60*(9), 513–515.

Weiss, D. W. (1988). Organ transplantation, medical ethics, and Jewish law. *Transplantation Proceedings, 20*(1, Suppl. 1), 1071–1075.

Wight, C. (1988). Organ procurement in Western Europe. *Transplantation Proceedings, 20*(1, Suppl. 1), 1003–1006.

Willis, R. W. (1988). Ethical issues involved in the use of anencephalics as organ donors. *Care Giver, 5*, 118–124.

Youngner, S. J., Landefeld, C. S., Coulton, C. J., Juknialis, B. W., & Leary, M. (1989). "Brain death" and organ retrieval: A cross-section survey of knowledge and concepts among health professionals. *Journal of the American Medical Association, 261*(15), 2206–2210.

Zaner, R. M. (1989). Anencephalics as organ donors. *Journal of Medicine and Philosophy, 14*(1), 61–78.

INDEX